Succeeding in Essays, Exams and OSCEs

for Nursing Students

Transforming Nursing Practice series

Transforming Nursing Practice is the first series of books designed to help students meet the requirements of the NMC Standards and Essential Skills Clusters for degree programmes. Each book addresses a core topic, and together they cover the generic knowledge required for all fields of practice.

Core knowledge titles:

Series editor: Dr Shirley Bach, Head of the School of Nursing and Midwifery at the University of Brighton

Personal and professional learning skills titles:

Series editors: Dr Mooi Standing, Independent Academic Consultant (UK and International) and Accredited NMC Reviewer and Dr Shirley Bach, Head of the School of Nursing and Midwifery at the University of Brighton

You can find more information on each of these titles and our other learning resources at **www.sagepub.co.uk**. Many of these titles are also available in various e-book formats; please visit our website for more information.

Succeeding in Essays, Exams and OSCEs

for Nursing Students

Kay Hutchfield
Mooi Standing

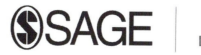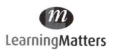

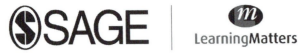

Learning Matters
An imprint of SAGE Publications Ltd
1 Oliver's Yard
55 City Road
London EC1Y 1SP

SAGE Publications Inc.
2455 Teller Road
Thousand Oaks, California 91320

SAGE Publications India Pvt Ltd
B 1/I 1 Mohan Cooperative Industrial Area
Mathura Road
New Delhi 110 044

SAGE Publications Asia-Pacific Pte Ltd
3 Church Street
#10-04 Samsung Hub
Singapore 049483

Editor: Becky Taylor
Development editor: Diana Chambers
Copy-editor: Amanda Crook
Production controller: Chris Marke
Project management: Diana Chambers
Marketing manager: Tamara Navaratnam
Cover design: Toucan Design
Typeset by: Kelly Winter
Printed by: TJ International LTD, Padstow, Cornwall

First published 2012

Library of Congress Control Number: 2012936250

British Library Cataloguing in Publication data

A catalogue record for this book is available from
the British Library

ISBN: 978 0 85725 827 4 (cloth)
ISBN: 978 0 85725 061 2 (paper)

Contents

Foreword

Succeeding in Essays, Exams and OSCEs for Nursing Students is an invaluable addition to the personal and professional learning skills titles in the *Transforming Nursing Practice* series. It takes the student reader on a guided journey in how to succeed in the variety of assessments they will undertake (written assignments, practice assessments, written examinations, portfolios, Objective Structured Clinical Examinations (OSCEs) and presentations) in order to become an NMC registered graduate nurse. An otherwise anxiety-provoking and dry topic is brought to life and made relevant to readers' needs using imaginative scenarios and creative activities to stimulate their involvement and understanding.

The book does not suggest that learning assessment skills is a substitute for being knowledgeable about nursing, but it does help readers to 'learn the knack' of knowing what specific aspects of theory and practice are being assessed and how to present a relevant response. This is important because knowing the answer is not sufficient to succeed unless students are able to communicate what they know. Readers will therefore find this book immensely helpful in preparing for and succeeding in their theoretical and practice assessments. It is written in a straightforward and engaging way, yet provides a comprehensive overview of how to succeed in all forms of assessments. Personal development is encouraged by stimulating readers' awareness of what they know or do not know, and how to address gaps in their subject knowledge or assessment technique. Professional development is facilitated as each chapter is clearly mapped to the relevant NMC standards of education and assessment, competencies and essential skills clusters. In this respect, the book conveys the importance of succeeding in assessments to demonstrate that nursing knowledge and skills are being applied to practice to benefit patients and other service users.

The skills used to succeed in assessments are also transferable to practise as a registered nurse. Nurses need to demonstrate their accountability not just by their actions but also their ability to articulate theoretical knowledge, logical reasoning and the evidence base supporting their actions. Hence, this book is not only invaluable to nursing students but also to nursing mentors and lecturers. I commend this book as essential reading for nursing students to enable them to show what they know by succeeding in assessments in order to qualify and practice as registered graduate nurses.

Dr Mooi Standing
Series Editor

About the authors

Kay Hutchfield began her nursing career in Oxford where she completed an orthopaedic nursing certificate. She then moved to London where she qualified as an adult nurse and worked in this field before undertaking a child nursing programme. She continued to work in this field before becoming a clinical teacher. On moving from London to Kent in 1986 she became a nurse teacher and has recently retired after 18 years as a senior lecturer in higher education. She has worked primarily in pre-registration nursing education, and has a keen interest in curriculum development. Kay has been programme director for three pre-registration child nursing programmes, and has developed a keen interest in developing students' fundamental research skills and managing risk in academic work as well as in care management.

Her experience working as a personal tutor and pathway director has provided her with the opportunity to see students both excel in and fail assessments. She has seen the negative impact that failing an assignment has on the student's confidence and ability to cope with their study workload. Some of the students who failed did so because they did not fully understand what was required of them, and others did not meet their own expectations, having worked hard but gained a mediocre mark.

Her first book in this series, *Information Skills for Nursing Students*, is designed to help students develop the skills of searching for literature that will provide the knowledge needed to register as a nurse. This book is designed to help students effectively demonstrate the knowledge they have gained in their nursing assessments and achieve their full potential.

Mooi Standing practised mental health and general nursing in various hospital and community settings before becoming a lecturer, and has been involved in nurse education for over 20 years. Mooi developed and continues to develop collaborative nursing, health studies and teaching programmes at undergraduate and post-qualifying levels on behalf of the International Nursing Colleges in Malaysia, and universities in Indonesia and the UK.

In addition, Mooi has taught and supervised students from undergraduate to PhD level in universities in the UK. She has established her professional and academic standing through her research studies on the perception of nursing and the development of clinical decision-making skills of nursing students. She has since developed and published a new critical framework for applying hermeneutic phenomenology, nine modes of practice on a cognitive continuum of decision-making, and a matrix on the perception of nursing and decision-making skills.

Mooi is an accredited Nursing and Midwifery Council (NMC, UK) reviewer who has applied her expertise and experience in approving, monitoring and assuring the quality of nursing programmes throughout the UK. She also provides external consultancy in curriculum development and quality assurance and enhancement, both nationally and internationally.

Pam Page is a senior lecturer at Anglia Ruskin University within the Acute Care Department. She is the pathway leader for the BSc (Hons) Acute Care and lectures across a range of acute care modules within pre- and post-registration nursing. Her clinical expertise is in acute and critical care nursing, and she is involved in developing OSCEs as a valid and effective learning, teaching and assessing method across nursing curricula. She is passionate about embedding theory into practice to enhance patient safety.

Acknowledgements

The authors wish to express their heartfelt thanks and gratitude to their respective spouses for their support and patience while this book was being written. We fully understand the frustration of putting family activities on hold and the surrender of common space while we were writing. Thank you all.

As always, it is a pleasure to work with the Learning Matters/SAGE production team in seeing this book to fruition.

Introduction

This book is designed to enable nursing students to understand how they can be successful in the range of assessments they will be required to complete on their nursing programme. The need to complete a range of different types of assessments is set out in nursing education standard 8 (NMC, 2010b) and all institutions providing nursing programmes are required to demonstrate this.

Standard 8: Assessment

R8.1   Programme providers must ensure that a variety of assessments are used to test the acquisition of approved outcomes, with reasonable adjustments for students with a disability.

R8.1.4 Programme providers must make it clear how service users and carers contribute to the assessment process.

R8.2   Programme providers must ensure that their assessment processes enable students to demonstrate fitness for practice and fitness for award.

R8.2.1 Programme providers must ensure that their assessment framework tests all programme outcomes.

Chapter 1 provides an introduction to the topic of assessment by exploring the purpose and process of assessment within pre-registration nursing programmes. It will enable you to understand the link between learning outcomes and your assessments through a series of activities linked to your own nursing programme. It also considers how formative feedback from tutors, peers, service users and mentors can be used effectively to enhance your performance in summative assessments.

Chapter 2 builds on the general introduction provided in Chapter 1 and your own previous experience of essay writing. It uses activities to work through the various stages of preparing for and then writing a successful written assessment. It includes the development of an assignment timeline in order to ensure that sufficient time is allowed to produce the quality of work required from a professional programme.

The focus of Chapters 3 and 5 is on assessment of practice in placements and through simulation. In Chapter 3 the focus is on making an effective plan for your placement to ensure a successful outcome. The importance of maximising practice learning opportunities is explored through the use of scenarios and activities, and emphasis is given to the importance of using the support available to ensure a successful practice assessment.

Success in examinations is the focus for Chapter 4, which begins by exploring how you can include the required level of critical analysis in examination answers. Your skills in planning a revision timetable and identifying ways of improving your examination performance are also developed through the use of activities and scenarios. The chapter concludes with consideration of the relevance of examination writing skills to nursing practice.

Chapter 5 explores the principles of producing a successful portfolio as well as considering how a portfolio can be used as a means of assessment. Producing a successful portfolio is explored through the use of scenarios and activities to increase your understanding of the demands of this type of assessment.

Chapter 6 is concerned with assessment using OSCEs (Objective Structured Clinical Examinations). This form of simulated practice assessment is common in nursing programmes. Scenarios are used to guide you in understanding how to prepare and participate successfully in OSCEs.

In Chapter 7 the focus is on success in presentations. This includes PowerPoint, poster and group presentations. Presentation skills are an essential skill for nurses, and this chapter explores some of the principles that will guide you to delivering a successful presentation.

The final short chapter draws together the support and resources available to you when undertaking assessments. It provides you with a quick reference point as it summarises the support and resources identified in the preceding chapters.

Chapter 1
An introduction to assessment in pre-registration nursing programmes

Kay Hutchfield

NMC Standards for Pre-registration Nursing Education

This chapter will address the following competencies:

Domain 2: Communication and interpersonal skills

8. All nurses must respect individual rights to confidentiality and keep information secure and confidential in accordance with the law and relevant ethical and regulatory frameworks, taking account of local protocols. They must also actively share personal information with others when the interests of safety and protection override the need for confidentiality.

Domain 3: Nursing practice and decision-making

1. All nurses must use up-to-date knowledge and evidence to assess, plan, deliver and evaluate care, communicate findings, influence change and promote health and best practice. They must make person-centred, evidence-based judgements and decisions, in partnership with others involved in the care process, to ensure high quality care. They must be able to recognise when the complexity of clinical decisions requires specialist knowledge and expertise, and consult or refer accordingly.

2. All nurses must possess a broad knowledge of the structure and functions of the human body, and other relevant knowledge from the life, behavioural and social sciences as applied to health, ill health, disability, ageing and death. They must have an in-depth knowledge of common physical and mental health problems and treatments in their own field of practice, including co-morbidity and physiological and psychological vulnerability.

Domain 4: Leadership, management and team working

4. All nurses must be self-aware and recognise how their own values, principles and assumptions may affect their practice. They must maintain their own personal and professional development, learning from experience, through supervision, feedback, reflection and evaluation.

Chapter aims

By the end of this chapter you should be able to:

- understand the purpose and process of the assessments on your nursing programme;
- understand the link between learning outcomes and your assessments;
- discuss the value of formative assessments;
- understand the role feedback plays in helping you improve your performance in assessment.

Introduction

Case study: Jenny

Jenny is a first-year nursing student and has been really enjoying her first year at university. She has made lots of new friends and joined several student union groups; she has a busy social life. She has attended university for her lectures and seminars but has found it difficult to fit independent study in around her university social life. She has not worried too much about her first assignments as she always managed to pass exams at school with some last-minute revision.

Six months into her programme Jenny goes to see her personal tutor as she has failed one of her first assignments and failed some competencies of her formative practice assessment. It is only at this point that she realises that if she does not pass her resubmitted course work, she will have to leave the programme. She also realises that if she fails her summative practice assessment she will have to repeat her practice assessment, which will result in her having to step off her programme for six months and rejoin with another student group. Jenny is distraught; she realises how important becoming a nurse is to her and that she will have to create a better balance between her studies and her social life if she is going to achieve her ambition. Jenny and her personal tutor develop an action plan that includes creating a study timetable, regular meetings with her personal tutor and support from the study resource centre in order to ensure that her resubmitted work is of an acceptable standard.

In 2010 the NMC published a *Strategic context report* (NMC, 2010a) that states:

> *Recent figures suggest attrition rates of around 28 per cent on pre-registration nursing courses.*
> (NMC, 2010a, para 36, p5)

This data suggests that over a quarter of nursing students fail to complete their nursing programme. There is a range of reasons for this high drop-out rate, but a proportion of those leaving will have done so because they have failed to pass all the assessment tasks they have been set. Jenny could have been one of those statistics as it is easy to put studying to one side when you start university as there are so many social activities happening that are fun and interesting.

Success in any nursing programme is dependent on the student passing a range of academic and practice assessments. Although normally students have at least one resit opportunity, having to repeat a practical assessment, resubmit a written assignment or resit an examination involves the student in additional work and stress on top of their normal study load.

This chapter is designed to enable you to understand how to prepare for your assessments and effectively address any assessment task. It will begin with some consideration of the meaning of assessment before discussing the concept of *fitness for practice and award*. A range of assessment methods will be explored to enable you to understand how you can best demonstrate your achievement of the standard required in practice and in your academic work. The chapter will explore the expectations of different levels of academic work and discuss how learning outcomes are linked to your academic and practice assessments in order to enable you to understand how to use this information to enhance your performance in assessments.

The purpose and process of assessment in pre-registration nursing programmes

To ensure that pre-registration nursing programmes produce nurses that are of quality and *fit for purpose*, the Nursing and Midwifery Council and the Quality Assurance Agency for Higher Education (QAA) have produced standards for assessment that need to be met to ensure that nursing students are fit for practice (NMC, 2010b) and award (QAA, 2006).

Your nursing programme will have been designed to meet the new standards for pre-registration nursing education (NMC, 2010b). This document also outlines the generic and pathway-specific competencies needed to meet the NMC requirements for registration as a nurse. Your university will have developed a programme based on these standards and will have been scrutinised by the NMC and the university's quality assurance processes to ensure that when you have successfully completed the programme you are *fit for practice and award*.

The assessment of practice will be explored in depth in Chapters 3 and 6. The next section will focus on explaining the concept of fitness for award.

Fitness for award

Your pre-registration nursing programme will have an exit award at a minimum of degree level. In higher education terms this is described as level 6 and is first-degree level. The Quality Assurance Agency has produced descriptors (QAA, 2008a) that outline the standard of academic work required for each level of a degree programme. If you are interested in learning more about these descriptors, go to the QAA framework for higher education qualifications (QAA, 2008a) available at www.qaa.ac.uk/Publications/InformationAndGuidance/Pages/The-framework-for-higher-education-qualifications-in-England-Wales-and-Northern-Ireland.aspx.

The assessments you undertake each year are designed to measure whether you have developed sufficiently to meet these academic criteria and progress to the next year. Your university will have developed assessment criteria that reflect those outlined by the QAA (2008a). When your work is assessed the marker will use these assessment criteria to award a mark depending on how well your work meets the criteria.

The QAA descriptors are designed for tutors rather than students, so you may find it easier to think about each year of your programme in the way outlined in the box.

Level	Expectation
4 (Year 1)	*Primarily descriptive* You will be expected to have read some core text from recommended academic books and journals, and be able to describe the core principles of the topic. Your knowledge must be accurate for safe practice and you must be able to demonstrate some emerging ability to analyse what you have read by making comparisons between literature and your experiences in practice. You may tend to make too much use of web-based resources rather than academic texts. You will be expected to write in a reasonable academic style, but some referencing errors will be anticipated. Writing at this level will gain you a pass at level 4, but for a really good mark you should aim to increase your level of reading and analysis as outlined in level 5.
5 (Year 2)	*Consistent analysis* You will be expected to have read more widely than at level 4, to have included in your reading some related current government/international policy, and to have a greater depth of understanding of the topic. This will increase your ability to compare and contrast the literature and research with your increased practice experience. You will begin to be more selective about the web-based material you use. Your academic writing style and reflective ability will need to be more advanced, with minimal referencing errors, and you should be able to write more concisely. Writing at this level will gain you a pass at level 5, but for a really good mark you should aim to increase your level of reading and critical analysis of primary sources of literature and research as outlined in level 6.
6 (Year 3)	*Critical analysis, evaluation and synthesis* You will be expected to read widely beyond recommended and core text, which should include predominately primary sources of literature, research and a range of relevant national and international policy documents. You should be able to analyse your topic at a more sophisticated level, supporting your arguments with evidence from research, academic literature and your increasing practice experience. You will be discriminating in your use of websites. In order to develop synthesis in your work you will need to be able to demonstrate your ability to make links between diverse sources to support the conclusions you have come to. You should be writing in a clear and concise academic style with only very minor errors in referencing if any.

Table 1.1: Expectations of undergraduate degree-level academic work

Each year of your programme will contain a number of course units or modules, the learning outcomes of which will be measured by an assessment.

In all new nursing programmes there are two progression points that occur around the end of years 1 and 2. At each progression point you will be required to have completed all your assessments of theory, practice and practice hours for the year.

Activity 1.1 — Critical thinking

Access your programme handbook and identify where the progression points fall. Read the section on assessment so that you are clear about your university's rules and regulations surrounding assessment and resubmissions.

As this answer is based on your own observation, there is no outline answer at the end of the chapter.

Your nursing programmes will have broad programme aims, and each module, unit or course within the three-year programme will have learning outcomes designed to support the achievement of the overall aims of the programme. These learning outcomes will also have been mapped against the standards (NMC, 2010b) and the QAA subject benchmark statements for nursing (QAA, 2008b) to ensure that your programme is fit for purpose. The learning outcomes for each course, unit or module must be clearly linked to the assessment task and practice experience to support the application of theory to practice.

Activity 1.2 — Critical thinking

Access your course/module handbook or the guide for the unit that you are currently undertaking. Find the learning outcomes for this course, module or unit and consider each of the following.

- How is each learning outcome measured in the assessment?
- Where can you find the marking criteria that the marker will use to assess your assignment?
- Are any of the outcomes assessed in practice?
- If so, how will these be assessed?
- At what academic level is the assignment being assessed?
- What number of academic credits will you gain for passing this assignment?

Now take a few moments to jot down what you have learnt that will help you tackle this assignment. Keep the notes you make on this exercise as we will return to it in Chapter 2.

Compare your notes to the ideas presented at the end of the chapter.

Generally, assessments will have both formative and summative elements. The next section will consider the difference between formative and summative assessment.

Formative and summative assessment

During your first year you will realise that many activities you engage in within university and practice settings are assessed informally (formatively) as well as formally (summatively) through course/module/unit and practice assessment. This can be seen as a form of continuous formative assessment that promotes knowledge and skills development in preparation for future formal, summative assessment. It is important that you actively participate in formative assessments throughout your three-year programme so that you gain a breadth of knowledge and under-standing and develop key skills such as team working and self-management.

Activity 1.3   *Reflection*

- Reflect back on your nursing programme so far and make a list of the activities that you have engaged in that have not been formally assessed but for which you have received some sort of feedback on your performance (informal or formative assessment).
- Once you have created your list, add to each entry what you think this activity was designed to help you learn or develop, using the table below.

Informally assessed activity	Personal and professional development

Once you have completed your table, go to the end of the chapter and see how well your ideas compare with the example given there.

Formative assessment may include a range of activities such as formative tests/self-testing, directed study, group presentations, oral presentations, debates and group scenario work. Feedback on your performance will not come just from your tutors, mentors and service users, but also through feedback from fellow students in the form of peer review. These types of formative assessment are designed to promote the development of the knowledge and skills you need to pass the associated summative assessment. It may also provide you with the opportunity to provide peer assessment to other students.

Summative assessments normally occur at the end of a module, course or unit of learning. You will be required to pass all summative assessments in order to progress on your nursing pro-gramme. The submission dates for summative assessments are very important, so look at the summative assessments you will be undertaking in the next year and put the dates in your diary.

The next section will consider the range of assessments that you may be expected to complete in order to demonstrate you have met the learning outcomes for the course, unit or module and be awarded academic credits.

Types of assessment that may be used to assess your professional knowledge

The NMC requires universities to ensure *that a variety of assessments are used to test the acquisition of approved outcomes* (NMC, 2010b, Standard 8). As a result, you will experience a range of assessments during your programme. The most common types of assessment are:

* coursework – essays and reports;
* examinations – seen and unseen, OSCE (Objective Structured Clinical Examination);
* practice-based assessments;
* portfolios of evidence;
* presentations – seminars and posters.

It is likely that you have a preference for a particular type of assessment; for example, you may prefer examinations to coursework, or practice-based assessment rather than written assessment. However, you will be required to pass a range of assessments, so it is important that you aim to improve your performance across all types.

Activity 1.4   *Decision-making*

This exercise may take you some time to complete but will be worth the effort when it comes to successfully completing your assessments.

1. Reflect on your experience of assessments so far and identify those you consider yourself good at and those you find particularly stressful.
2. Look through your student handbook and make a list of the assessments you are going to be faced with in the next year. The assessments should be listed in order of their submission dates. Are there any assessments types that you have not experienced before?
3. Using your lists, make a plan for working through the chapters of this book most relevant to you. Begin with assignment types that you have never encountered before or those where you lack confidence. In this way you can make the most of your efforts in your assessments.

For some idea of what such a plan might look like, go to the end of the chapter and look under Activity 1.4.

The role feedback has in the assessment process and how to utilise it successfully

Let's return to Jenny, the nursing student we met at the beginning of this chapter, and consider how formative assessment and feedback can help Jenny with her failed assessments. First, we will consider the failed competencies in practice. These all related to professional behaviour and the manner in which Jenny presented herself in practice. We will begin looking at this from Jenny's perspective.

Case study: Jenny's perspective

Jenny was on her first ward placement and was really enjoying it, but she found it difficult getting up early in the morning and had been late for shifts on two occasions. She thought her mentor had made an unnecessary fuss as she was only five minutes late. Her mentor had also 'moaned at her' for not having a pen and had refused to let her wear her wristwatch, making her pin it inside her tunic pocket. When her formative assessment was being arranged, it came as a real shock to Jenny when her mentor, Sarah, told her she had asked the link tutor for the placement to come to the assessment as it was likely she would fail some competencies.

Mentor's perspective

Sarah is an experienced nurse, mentor and sign-off mentor. Jenny was one of many first-year students Sarah had mentored, and she saw it as very important that new students understood their professional responsibilities. Jenny was a lively student who was popular with the elderly patients on her ward; she was quick to pick up new skills and was keen to learn. However, there were two problems: Jenny's timekeeping and her preparation for work. Jenny had been late for her shift on two occasions and on several occasions had arrived for work without a pen and wearing her wristwatch on her arm. Despite talking to Jenny several times about this behaviour she felt Jenny thought she was making a 'fuss about nothing'. She felt she was left with no option but to fail Jenny for some of the competencies of her formative practice assessment, so she telephoned the link teacher to ask her to attend the meeting between herself and Jenny.

This situation is a difficult one for all involved and will be explored further in the chapter on practice assessment. For the moment we will focus on what formative feedback Jenny could have responded to that might have enabled her to avoid this situation and for her to have developed a more positive relationship with her mentor.

First, let's consider the positive formative feedback Jenny had received. She was popular with the patients; she knew this because they told her how kind she was and that she was *such a good nurse*. One of the relatives had given her a card thanking her for the care she had given her father. On the basis of user and carer feedback Jenny felt she was doing well.

When working with her mentor in direct patient care Jenny had also had a lot of positive feedback from her mentor. She had had the opportunity to develop new skills under supervision and had benefited from discussing the patient's conditions with her mentor. Her mentor was good at praising her when she completed tasks successfully, and as a result of this positive feedback she felt she was developing in competence and confidence in some fundamental areas of patient care.

This positive feedback gave Jenny some confidence, so perhaps this was why she was rather dismissive about the feedback on her punctuality and presentation at work. The activity below provides you with the opportunity to consider what action Jenny might have taken.

Activity 1.5   *Critical thinking*

Imagine you are Jenny. How did Jenny manage to misinterpret the significance of the negative feedback she had been given? What questions might you have asked the mentor in order to understand her concerns about Jenny's behaviour? *Jot down your questions and then refer to the suggested questions and possible responses made at the end of the chapter.*

This activity was intended to highlight the importance of responding to negative feedback in a positive and proactive way, and recognise the danger of dismissing it as unimportant. It can sometimes be quite challenging to accept criticism, but as long as it is constructive, this type of feedback will enable you to understand yourself better, and if responded to appropriately, will promote your professional development. If you are able to respond positively to formative feedback, then you will increase your chances of being successful in your summative assessment.

We discussed how summative assessments have to be achieved by a specific point in a programme. Feedback from these assessments is crucially important if you are going to be able to demonstrate progression and continuing academic and professional development in theory and practice. Summative assessment feedback will be returned to in the chapters on essays and practice assessment.

Chapter summary

Looking back over this chapter you should now have a clear understanding of the purpose of assessment within your pre-registration programme and the range of assessments that you are likely to encounter. You will be clear about how formative assessment contributes to the summative assessment of your programme and demonstration of the achievement of the learning outcomes. In addition, you will begin to understand how to use assessment feedback to improve your performance in assessment and have a plan for using the content of this book in a way that is most suited to your needs.

Activities: brief outline answers

Activity 1.2: Critical thinking (page 7)

What I have learnt from considering the learning outcomes:

- The content I need to include in my assignment and what will be assessed in practice.
- The academic level I need to achieve and the criteria that will be used to mark my work.
- The level of reading, knowledge and analysis I need to demonstrate in order to gain the grade I would like.
- The links with learning in practice.
- The academic credits awarded for my assessment.

Activity 1.3: Reflection (page 8)

Informally assessed activity	Personal and professional development
Group presentation	Knowledge of topic, learnt about group dynamics and working in a team, communication, use of PowerPoint.
Personal tutor meetings	Feedback on and development of personal development plans and learning contracts.
Discussion/debate	Enhanced ability to listen, clearly presenting my views, increasing confidence in expressing my views, recognition of other perspectives on a topic.
Practice	Service user feedback and mentor feedback on progress in achieving aims of learning contract and practice competencies each shift.

Activity 1.4: Decision-making

Your plan might look something like this.

OSCE in six weeks	Read chapter on OSCE in next two weeks and incorporate ideas into plan. Find out when preparation sessions are and what opportunities there are to practise skills prior to OSCE.
Case study in four weeks	Confident with this. Submit plan next week to tutor. Book in to an advanced library searching session to access more advanced literature/research.
Practice assessment in seven weeks	Read chapter on practice assessment once case study submitted, and complete a draft learning contract after OSCE.
Group formative presentation in eight weeks	Did not enjoy last presentation as group did not work together well. Need to read chapter on presentations and incorporate ideas into my plan. Discuss with personal tutor how I might have a positive influence on group dynamics this time around.

An introduction to assessment

Activity 1.5: Critical thinking (page 11)

Below are some possible questions and answers that might have enabled Jenny to understand the mentor's perspective and why it was so important to understand the need to change her behaviour.

Jenny: You were obviously really cross with me this morning but I was only five minutes late. Why were you so angry?

Sarah: In nursing you have to work as a team, and the night shift had had a really busy night. It is important that the day shift turn up on time so that night staff can finish their shift on time. It's about being professional. You just turned up late and didn't seem to realise that this is not what team work is about. Also, you did not phone in to say that you would be late. That reflected badly on me – like I wasn't doing my job as your mentor. The night staff were asking me where you were and I had no answer.

Jenny: I know I forgot to put my watch in my tunic pocket or bring a pen this morning but why is this so important?

Sarah: In your orientation to the ward it was made quite clear that you must arrive on duty fit for work. Wearing a wristwatch contravenes the trust infection control policy and the university uniform policy. As your mentor I am accountable for your actions, and wearing a wristwatch puts patients at risk from cross-infection and physical harm, so I have a duty to raise these issues with you. In terms of the pen, you know how important it is to write down observations and nursing interventions as you undertake them, and you cannot be running around borrowing pens from other members of staff. You need to arrive on duty ready for work.

Further reading

NMC (2011a) *Guidance for students*. Available at: **www.nmc-uk.org/Students/Guidance-for-students/**.

If Jenny had been familiar with the Nursing and Midwifery Council's guidance for student nurses, she might have been more aware of the behaviour expected of her by her mentor. Make sure you are familiar with the content of this document.

Goodman, B and Clemow, R (2010) *Nursing and collaborative practice*. Exeter: Learning Matters.

This book provides some useful guidance and professional perspectives on working collaboratively with others.

Griffiths, R and Tengriah, C (2010) *Law and professional issues in nursing people*. Exeter: Learning Matters.

Chapter 12, on confidentiality, will enable you to fully understand your responsibilities in maintaining confidentiality in your assessments and in your practice.

Useful websites

http://standards.nmc-uk.org/PreRegNursing/statutory/background/Pages/Background-and-Context.aspx

The new NMC standards for pre-registration nursing education are available through this link. The most relevant aspects for you to be aware of are the generic and field competencies, which are in Section 2, and the essential skills clusters in the Annexe section.

If you are interested in the standards and benchmarks that govern your university course, details can be found on the QAA website. Some of the useful links are listed below

www.qaa.ac.uk/AssuringStandardsAndQuality/academic-credit/Pages/default.aspx

The Quality Assurance Agency website offers more information on academic credits.

www.qaa.ac.uk/Publications/InformationAndGuidance/Pages/understanding-assessment.aspx

The purpose of the QAA guide *Understanding assessment: its role in safeguarding academic standards and quality in higher education* is to help staff involved in assessment in higher education to use assessment effectively, as a means of maintaining both the academic standards of taught awards and ensuring and enhancing the quality of the student learning experience.

Access your university home page and search for the quality assurance site. From there find the regulations your university has developed on assessment. This may be useful to you in the future if you need to know what the university assessment regulations are.

Chapter 2
Succeeding in written assignments

Kay Hutchfield

NMC Standards for Pre-registration Nursing Education

This chapter will address the following competencies:

Domain 1: Professional values

9. All nurses must appreciate the value of evidence in practice, be able to understand and appraise research, apply relevant theory and research findings to their work, and identify areas for further investigation.

Domain 2: Communication and interpersonal skills

3. All nurses must use the full range of communication methods, including verbal, non-verbal and written, to acquire, interpret and record their knowledge and understanding of people's needs. They must be aware of their own values and beliefs and the impact this may have on their communication with others. They must take account of the many different ways people communicate and how these may be influenced by ill health, disability and other factors, and be able to recognise and respond effectively when a person finds it hard to communicate.

Domain 3: Nursing practice and decision-making

2. All nurses must possess a broad knowledge of the structure and functions of the human body, and other relevant knowledge from the life, behavioural and social sciences as applied to health, ill health, disability, ageing and death. They must have an in-depth knowledge of common physical and mental health problems and treatments in their own field of practice, including co-morbidity and physiological and psychological vulnerability.

NMC Essential Skills Clusters

This chapter will address the following ESCs:

Cluster: Care, compassion and communication

1. As partners in the care process, people can trust a newly registered graduate nurse to provide collaborative care based on the highest standards, knowledge and competence.
6. People can trust the newly registered graduate nurse to engage therapeutically and actively listen to their needs and concerns, responding using skills that are helpful, providing information that is clear, accurate, meaningful and free from jargon.
7. People can trust the newly registered graduate nurse to protect and keep as confidential all information relating to them.

Introduction

This chapter will introduce you to the processes you need to complete in order to successfully plan and construct a written assignment. This type of assignment may take the form of an essay or a similar task such as writing a case study or a report. The generic principles discussed here will also have relevance to other forms of assignment explored in later chapters, and will be particularly important to you in your final extended piece of work, e.g. your dissertation.

You will be encouraged to reflect on your current experience of essay writing and how this may be developed into a sound academic style as required by your university. It is anticipated that you have achieved the minimum university entry requirement of English language equivalent to a Grade C at GCSE. If this is not the case or you have had any concerns regarding sentence construction, spelling or paragraphing in the past, then it is important that you take action now. Your university will have a student study support centre where you will be able to access support and resources. In addition, there are some excellent books and websites that can help, and they are listed at the end of this chapter.

Activity 2.1 — *Reflection*

Take a moment to reflect on your experience of writing essays or reports, and jot down those things you are confident in as well as those areas where you know you need to improve. When you've completed your list, access your university website and locate the study support centre. Look at the support they offer that will help you develop your writing skills. For example, there may be workshops available on essay writing and revising for examinations or resources on how to write critically. Alternatively, you may feel that attending an introduction to referencing would be more useful. It all depends on what is the most relevant for you. If you are familiar with the resources your student study support centre has to offer and know how to access them, then you will know where to go for help should the need arise.

As this activity is based on your own reflection, there is no outline answer at the end of the chapter.

In Chapter 1 you were introduced to Jenny, a first-year nursing student who had failed an assignment. In this chapter we will look at some of the reasons why Jenny was unsuccessful and consider a second-year student and a third-year student as they develop their academic skills in order to progress through their nursing programme.

Case study: Jenny

Jenny was used to succeeding at school with some last-minute work, so she was shocked to find herself failing her first academic assignment at university. Her first reaction was panic as she realised that other students that she thought less able than herself had passed – some with very good marks. She was embarrassed by her failure and at first tried to pretend that it really was 'no big deal', but when she met with her personal tutor she realised that she needed to put some real effort into her resubmission if she was to pass and remain on the programme.

You probably already have some ideas on how Jenny could have avoided failing her first assignment. The following activity provides you with the opportunity to formalise those thoughts.

Activity 2.2   *Critical thinking*

Take a moment to think about how you might feel if you were in Jenny's shoes, and then answer the following questions.

- What action might Jenny have taken to avoid failing her assignment?
- How will Jenny know what she has done wrong?
- What action can Jenny take to ensure her resubmission is likely to be successful?

Make a note of your answers as we will return to them again at the end of the next section.

This chapter will continue by exploring how Jenny could have worked in order to avoid failing her assignment before discussing what Jenny needs to do now to understand the mistakes she made with her first submission. This will include discussion on how to make the maximum use of the help and support available for her resubmission. The chapter will conclude with an exploration of the various types of written assignments and the specific requirements they each demand.

- What action might Jenny have taken to avoid failing her assignment?

There are generic activities that Jenny could have completed to ensure her assignment was of a satisfactory standard. Such actions can be applied to all assignments and will be explored under the headings of preparation, writing the assignment and learning from feedback. Each of these will be considered in turn before moving on to the next question in Activity 2.2.

Preparation

This section is called preparation rather than just making a plan, as there are several elements to successful preparation that will be presented as a series of steps.

Step 1: What format of written assignment is required?

The first step in any assignment preparation is understanding the way in which the assignment needs to be presented. This information should be evident from the assessment title and guidelines in your module, course or unit handbook. Below are some examples.

- *Year 1 assessment*: a report that outlines the findings of a community profiling exercise and makes recommendations for the improvement of the health of a specific community group with reference to specific social policy (2,000 words).
- *Year 2 assessment*: a 3,000-word reflective essay that analyses your academic progression and professional development during the first and second year of your nursing programme.
- *Year 3 assessment*: a case study that provides a rationale for the care delivered to a client and critically evaluates the nursing care provided (3,000 words).

You will notice that each assignment has an associated word allowance. Normally, students are allowed to submit an assignment that is 10 per cent under or over this word allowance. This is to ensure that you submit enough information on the subject to assess whether you have gained sufficient understanding for safe practice, and to assess your ability to communicate information clearly and concisely. You are likely to be penalised if you exceed the word allowance. If your written assignment is less than the minimum word allowance, you are unlikely to have understood the subject at sufficient depth to gain a pass.

The assessment title also provides details of the format required. Table 2.1 outlines what is likely to be required from the five most common written assignments.

Type of written assignment	Specific considerations
An essay	An academic essay is normally written in prose with no headings, sub-headings, lists or bullet points. It is normally written in the third person (objective tense) and must be supported with reference to published literature and research. The reference list comes at the end of the essay, and any lists or diagrams are normally in an appendix after the reference list. Appendices and the reference list are not included in the word allowance. Appendices should contain supporting evidence only (for example, in the form of a genogram) and not used as a means of expanding the word allowance.

Table 2.1: Written assignment formats

Type of written assignment	Specific considerations
A report or research critique/study	In this type of written assignment it is usual to use headings and sub-headings and to include figures, graphs and diagrams within the text of the written report. It is likely that your module/course/unit handbook will provide you with guidance on the headings that need to be included. A report is normally written in the third person.
A reflective essay	This type of written assignment requires you to reflect on your experiences, and you may be required to write in the first person as you are recounting a personal experience. It is important to use a model of reflection to inform your work. This will allow you to demonstrate that you understand the process of reflection and will also provide a structure to your assignment. When you are reflecting on your practice experiences you must be careful to maintain the confidentiality of your mentor, other professional colleagues and their workplace as well as the patient or client. You need to use generic terms, e.g. w*hile on a community placement, my mentor, a community physician.* Another book in this series, *Reflective practice in nursing* (Howatson-Jones, 2010), provides a very useful introduction to a range of models of reflection from which you can select one that suits you.
A case study	This type of written assignment is focused on a specific patient or group of clients you have cared for. You will need to seek permission from the patient or client to use health information about them in your essay. Some institutions require you to have written permission before you can use this information in your work. It is important you gain this permission *before* you begin your essay. In this type of assignment it is essential that you respect the confidentiality of the person whose information you propose to use, so you must not use their real name. Try to avoid impersonal pseudonyms such as patient X but rather an alternative name that cannot be linked to the patient, such as Mr Smith.

Table 2.1: Continued

Type of written assignment	Specific considerations
Dissertation/ Individual Study	In this type of written assignment you must link theory to the patient experience and nursing interventions to introduce synthesis into your work and gain a good mark. This type of written assignment is usually a larger piece of work submitted towards the end of your programme. You will be provided with clear guidelines in your module/course/unit handbook in terms of the use of headings, sub-headings, graphs, etc. You will also be provided with supervision and guidance from an academic tutor. In these types of written assignment the reference list is likely to be extensive.

Table 2.1: Continued

If you present your written assignment in the wrong format, then you are likely to be penalised and so lose marks. Make sure you read the assignment guidelines carefully and seek clarification from your module/course or unit leader if you are still unclear.

At this stage you should also check the word allowance and whether any figures and tables are included in the word allowance to avoid accidentally exceeding the word allowance.

Activity 2.3   *Critical thinking*

- Access your programme/course handbook and find an overview of the assessments.
- Identify all the written assignments you will need to complete and make a note of the format required for future reference.
- Identify the next written assignment you are required to complete for one year and create an electronic template in Word based on the guidelines provided. Insert the assessment title on the front page along with the word allowance. Insert page numbers. Ensure that you use the correct line spacing; include any headings and appendices indicated in the assignment guidelines and insert a space for your reference list before any appendices.
- Save your template ready to begin your assignment.

As this answer is based on your own assignment, there is no outline answer at the end of the chapter.

Having created the format for your written assignment, we move on to the second step in the preparation process; deciding what content to include.

Step 2: What content do I include in my written assignment?

In Chapter 1 we discussed the link between learning outcomes and assessments, so your module/course or unit handbook should be your first port of call when deciding what content you need to cover in your written assignment. For the next activity you will need to have the module/course or unit handbook for your next written assignment, a folder, notepaper and access to your module/course/unit learning resources, which may be provided electronically via your university virtual learning environment (VLE).

Activity 2.4   *Critical thinking*

- Examine the learning outcomes and decide what knowledge these are asking you to demonstrate in your written assignment and note them down in a list.
- Check the module content and add any additional content that may be included there.
- Access the teaching resources associated with the module/course or unit (e.g. VLE) and add any additional content you have identified.
- Gather all this information with your module/course/unit handbook in a folder/ring binder.

As this answer is based on your own experience, there is no outline answer at the end of the chapter.

You now have a comprehensive list of the content you need to include in your assignment and are ready to progress to the next stage; understanding the topic.

Step 3: Understanding the topic of written assignment

Your list of content marks the beginning of a very important stage in the preparation for writing your assignment.

- *Attending lectures and seminars* These will play a key part in understanding the module, course or unit content as they provide you with the opportunity to ask questions and seek clarification.
- *Accessing and reading relevant sections of the core texts* You will find core text listed in your module/course/unit handbook and accessing them is an important step in understanding the topic. Use the learning outcomes and the Contents page of core text to select the most relevant sections of core text to read. It is advisable to access the library early to reserve any core texts, as you may find that you will have to wait for them to become available.
- *Seeking additional information* As you progress to your second and third year you will be expected to read more widely and be discriminating in your use of web-based information. You will be expected to become increasingly active in seeking additional information that will help you understand the topic and develop depth to your understanding. This will allow you to be more critical and effective in your evaluation and appraisal of the literature and related practice experiences.

Activity 2.5   *Reflection*

In the section above it is evident that as you progress through your programme you will be increasingly expected to extend the range of material you read in preparation for any assignment. We recommend you access another book in this series, *Information skills for nursing students* (Hutchfield, 2010).

- Complete the exercises at the end of Chapters 2 and 3 of that book.
- Identify any areas you need to revisit in these chapters to develop your skills.
- Access the library page of your university website and find the resources provided to help improve your library skills. These may include library workshops as well as online resources.

The answer to this activity is contained within the book Information skills for nursing students, *so there is no answer at the end of this chapter.*

With sound information-searching skills you can gather together the information you need for your assignment and be in a position to create an assignment plan and timeline.

Step 4: Planning a written assignment and developing a timeline

Any assignment will have a submission date. You must meet this deadline or it will count as a failed first attempt. Another consequence of a failed assignment is that any resubmission is normally capped at the pass mark (e.g. 40%), even if the work is of good quality. A low mark like this can affect your overall average mark and impact on your final award classification. Therefore, it is a good idea to enter assignment submission dates into your diary so that you do not accidentally miss these deadlines.

When planning an assignment timeline it is important to work backwards from the assignment submission date so that you plan in sufficient time to find and read the information you need to understand the topic before you start to write.

Table 2.2 is an example of an assignment timeline spread over an eight-week period. Using an assignment timeline can be particularly important when you have a number of different assessments due within a short space of time. Making a timeline that includes all these assessments as well as any important social events you need to accommodate is an important process in the achievement of a successful outcome for all your assessments.

Activity 2.6   *Critical thinking*

Use the assessment you identified earlier in Activity 2.4.

- Create your own assignment timeline.
- Build in to it any other deadlines or practice placements you may have that overlap with this assignment and for which you may need to make adjustments.

continued . . .

Week								Submit assignment
1	2	3	4	5	6	7	8	
Read module handbook and make an initial list of content.	Create an assignment template and draft the introduction based on assignment title/ question. Reserve core textbooks. Start reference list.	Read and make notes on core material and learning resources. Add to reference list.	Plan assignment structure and order of content and discuss with tutor.	Begin first draft of assignment. Use list of content to search the library resources for additional information.	More reading and making notes on material accessed.	Complete first draft, reference list and any appendices. Final search for any additional material required.	Review assignment against learning outcomes, content and assignment guide, then complete final draft.	

Table 2.2: Timeline

continued . . .

- Build a detailed weekly timetable that identifies the specific dates work is going to be undertaken.
- Once you have submitted your assignment, return to your plan and evaluate how effectively it reflected what you actually did.
- Build any improvements needed in to your next assignment timeline.
- When you receive the results of your assignment, revisit your timeline and identify any additional areas for improvement.

As this answer is based on your own experience, there is no outline answer at the end of the chapter.

Creating an essay plan

Much has been written about how to structure written assignments, and a range of recommended texts are provided at the end of this chapter if you wish to read more widely on the topic. In principle, all written assignments have at least three elements: an introduction, a main body and a conclusion, plus a reference list.

Before looking at each of these sections in the table on p23, we will take a moment to consider the assignment question or task. It seems obvious to state how important it is to answer the question or task set if you wish to be successful in your assessments. Unfortunately, it is not uncommon for students to change the title of an assignment and, as a consequence, fail to meet the assignment task.

Case study: Lucy

Lucy is a third-year student who has just completed her first piece of work at level 6. The assessment was: 'A case study that provides a rationale for the care delivered to a client and critically evaluates the nursing care provided (3,000 words)'.

Lucy had discussed this assignment with her mentor and had gained permission from the parents of a newly diagnosed diabetic child to use their child as her case study. She had found the subject of diabetes fascinating and had spent a lot of time with the diabetic specialist nurse extending her knowledge of the subject. She had also read widely on the topic and enjoyed writing the assignment.

However, Lucy gave her assignment the title 'Managing childhood diabetes'. Although she mentioned the child in her introduction and respected patient confidentiality, this was the only time she really mentioned the child. She wrote a very generic essay on childhood diabetes rather than a focused assignment that provided an evidenced-based rationale for the treatment the child received. As there was no real focus on the child's experience Lucy also failed to evaluate the nursing interventions the child received. Although Lucy had submitted a well-researched assignment on childhood diabetes, it did not meet the learning outcomes for this assessment.

Imagine Lucy's disappointment when she learnt that she had failed this assessment.

In order to avoid the mistake Lucy made, make sure the assigned assignment title features at the beginning of your work and is accurately reflected in your introduction, content and conclusion. If you change the title of the assignment, you will change the focus. Changing the focus is likely to result in failing the assessment.

The next section will consider the structure of written assessments. A sound logical structure (see Table 2.3 below) will help the person marking your work to follow your reasoning and arguments, and is likely to result in a successful assessment.

Now that you have completed your preparation, you are in the position to return to the first question in Activity 2.2. Revisit the answer you noted down and add any other actions Jenny could have taken to minimise her risk of failure. Compare your list with those at the end of the chapter.

Introduction	An introduction should be brief and outline what will be included and how the assignment question/task will be addressed. It will include any relevant definitions and may make reference to how confidentiality is maintained if you are making reference to practice placement, practice colleagues or patients/clients.
Main body	This section should reflect the key aspects you wish to explore. You may find that when you have written each section you will need to adjust the sequence of the content so that one section flows logically into the next. If you are writing a report or critique, you may be provided with headings that should structure this section.
	Make sure that your introduction reflects the order in which you present the information in the main body and that you have not strayed from the main purpose of the assignment.
	Discussion in this section must make reference to published academic/professional literature and research.
Conclusion	Your conclusion will draw together the discussion you have had in the main body and present some conclusions based on the evidence you have presented. You should not introduce any new material or references in this section.

Table 2.3: Assignment structure

Writing your assignment

This stage of assignment writing will also be divided into steps in order to consider the various aspects involved.

Step 1: Writing style

Assignments are normally written in the third person unless otherwise stated in the assignment guidelines. This formal approach to writing is the same you will see in professional journals and research papers. Using this style will hopefully encourage you to examine a topic from different perspectives and challenge your own perceptions though greater understanding.

If you are new to writing in the third person, try the example in Activity 2.7.

Activity 2.7   *Critical thinking*

Below is an example written in the first person (subjective tense):

> *When I was on a placement on a surgical ward I met a really nice woman who had been told she had cancer. She was obviously very upset and I didn't know what to say so went to find my mentor for help.*

Rewrite the example in the third person and academic style.

Check your answer with the one provided at the end of the chapter.

Step 2: Demonstrating what you know

It is important at this stage that you select from the material you have read the most relevant material to the topic of the assignment. This is necessary if you are to produce a focused and concise piece of work. This can sometimes be difficult if, like Lucy, you find a particular aspect really interesting. However, if it is not directly linked to the assignment, you should not include it, no matter how interesting. When you find yourself in this situation, just accept that you have developed a wider insight into the topic that will enhance your practice in the future rather than add irrelevant information to your assignment. This is where Lucy went wrong with her case study.

Writing concisely is also an important skill to develop for practice as well as for your academic work. As you read, group similar ideas found in different literature together as well as any counter-arguments, so you demonstrate your breadth of reading and your ability to synthesise information into a concise statement.

Case study: Mark

Mark is a mature second-year student. He has opted for a career change after seven years in the print industry and really wants to make a success of a career in mental health nursing. He studies hard and enjoys reading around the topics he has to study, but when it comes to writing the assignment he quickly runs out of words. He is worried as, despite working hard, he has only achieved mediocre marks in his first year and is anxious that he will not be able to pass his written assignments in Year 2.

---

continued . . .

Feedback from two of his written assignments state that he has a tendency to write in a bullet point/list fashion that makes his work hard to read. *Mark is not sure what this means and has made an appointment to see his personal tutor who has asked him to bring his Year 1 written assignments with him.*

At the meeting his tutor quickly identifies that Mark is including relevant content from a good range of literature but is listing rather than integrating and discussing what he has read. For example, in one assignment he has described five definitions of mental health and discussed them all separately, using up a large amount of his word allowance in his introduction. His tutor suggested he could still use the material but in a more concise manner. For example:

A number of definitions of mental health exist (Smith, 2011, James, 2009, DoH, 2008, WHO, 2007). For the purpose of this assignment the WHO definition will be used as it . . .

From this experience Mark was able to develop a more concise way of writing yet still demonstrate the breadth of reading he had undertaken. This also left him with more words to show his depth of understanding and begin to develop analysis and critical evaluation in his written assignments.

Step 3: Writing critically

For each year of your programme there will be a minimum level you will have to achieve in terms of your knowledge base and critical thinking ability. In order to demonstrate that you have an adequate knowledge base for safe practice you will need to use evidence in the form of research, NICE guidelines, social policy and professional literature to support your work as well as demonstrating insight into the perspective of the service user through service user organisations, research and blogs.

In order to develop your critical writing skills you will need to read critically so that as you read you begin to question the arguments the literature puts forward and consider the quality of the evidence you are accessing. Compare what you are reading to your experience in practice and explore the challenges faced when implementing theory in practice.

When you begin to write, remember the questions you were asking yourself and develop them into statements that can illustrate your critical thinking ability. For example, use statements that include:

- this view can be challenged because . . .
- this would suggest . . .
- when implementing this policy in practice challenges emerge such as . . .
- practice experience suggests that the client perspective is not always taken into account. For example . . ..

To achieve the required level of critical discussion, take note of the words used in the assignment question/title. Use Table 2.4 to ensure that you understand the type of discussion you need to introduce into your essay.

Analyse	Consider in detail the subject through reading relevant literature so that you can identify essential features or meaning.
Compare	Explore subjects/issues to discover both the similarities and differences between them.
Contrast	Identify a difference between two or more things that is evident when they are compared.
Critically	Read sufficiently to be able to offer a critique/evaluation by examining and judging something, carefully using the literature and/or practice experience.
Debate	Discuss by involving opposing viewpoints often linked to ethical issues such as consent, treatment options or end-of-life care.
Define	Use appropriate literature to identify the meaning of a word, phrase etc. It is likely to lead on to ask you to analyse or evaluate something. For example, define mental health and discuss the role the nurse can play in promoting mental health within a specific context.
Describe	Describe or give an account of what has been written about a specific subject, giving an accurate interpretation of what you have read.
Develop	Use a range of literature to elaborate or expand in detail on a subject, idea or statement.
Discuss	Consider or examine a subject using argument and comment that reflects the content of relevant literature and practice experience.
Distinguish	Identify and explore the difference between subjects: for example, with reference to the literature distinguish between the concepts of respite care, palliative care and end-of-life care.
Evaluate	Make a judgement on the value, quality or significance of something; for example, using the literature, social policy and examples from practice, evaluate the quality of nursing care delivered to an elderly patient.
Examine	Similar to analyse. Inspect or scrutinise carefully.
Explain	Similar to describe. Give an explanation.
Explore	Similar to discuss and examine. Look into closely.
Interpret	Similar to describe. Provide an explanation of the meaning of a subject/concept supported with reference to relevant literature.
Justify	Use literature and practice experience to defend or uphold actual/proposed action.

Table 2.4: Commonly used key words in essay titles

Step 4: Avoiding plagiarism

Throughout this chapter reference has been made to the importance of understanding your assignment topic or task through relevant reading. However, you must avoid copying sections of the literature you have read into your essay. If you do this without making reference to the author of the literature, you will find yourself accused of plagiarism, which, in serious cases, can result in you being asked to leave the programme.

Plagiarism is concerned with cheating and presenting the work of others as your own. In a profession such as nursing, cheating of any kind is taken very seriously as it raises questions about the integrity and suitability of the student for entry to the nursing profession.

Plagiarism includes direct copying of published work, and copying, accessing or purchasing on the internet the work of someone else and presenting it as your own. Plagiarism also applies if you submit some of your own work that has already been awarded a mark as part of another assignment.

Universities now tend to use plagiarism software to check student assignments for evidence of plagiarism. However, even if such software is not used in your university, you must remember that those marking your work will be experts in the field and will be familiar with the literature associated with the topic, so they will routinely identify cases of plagiarism without the aid of computer software.

The best way to avoid plagiarism is to make detailed notes as you read the literature so that you are paraphrasing (summarising and putting in your own words) what you have read as you go along. As part of this note-taking process you can identify any definitions or key points that you may wish to use as direct quotes. Remember to make a note of page numbers for any direct quotes you may need to use.

Learning from feedback

We have already touched on how feedback can be used to improve performance. Now we will move on to consider this further under the question:

• How will Jenny know what she has done wrong?

The feedback received from the tutor who marked her work is the most important information Jenny needs to understand and act upon in order to pass her resubmitted assessment. The tutor who marked the first submission may mark the resubmission, so it is important that Jenny takes notice of the comments the marker has made on her work.

Activity 2.8   *Decision-making*

Below is a copy of the feedback on Jenny's assignment.

This assignment contains some interesting information; however, most of the content addresses learning outcome 2 and 3, and pays scant attention to learning outcome 1, which requires you to demonstrate your understanding of the concept of caring.

It is presented in report rather than essay format, and the use of bullet points is not appropriate for an academic essay. In places your use of academic writing style is poor, e.g. on page 4 you have written I think it is really important that nurses are kind and caring. *This is a subjective comment and needs to be supported with reference to published work. For example, quality nursing care has been described as* meeting human needs through caring, empathetic, respectful interactions within which responsibility, intentionality and advocacy form an essential, integral foundation *(Burhans and Alligood, p1689).*

You have used only one of the core texts to support your work, but you needed to read more widely as there is a tendency to over-rely on this one text and on dubious web-based information such as .com sources rather than use a range of core texts and more reliable sites such as the Department of Health site at dh.gov.uk. Remember to make maximum use of the core texts contained within the module bibliography. Use of more of this core material would have enhanced your work.

Some attempt is made to write in an academic style but many statements are unsupported with a reference and the reference list contains many errors. You have a tendency to present facts descriptively with limited attempts to compare or contrast information from a range of sources.

Please contact me for tutorial support for your resubmission.

Return to your notes on Activity 2.2. What can you add to your list now that you have read Jenny's feedback? Compare your answer to the illustrative answer to Activity 2.2 at the end of the chapter. Put yourself in Jenny's shoes. How would you approach this resubmission?

In addition to this written feedback, Jenny has been offered additional feedback at a meeting with the marker of her work. It is important that Jenny takes up this offer to ensure she has fully understood the written feedback and is clear about what she needs to do to improve her first submission. It is important she prepares properly for this meeting by taking with her a copy of her assignment, the feedback and the module/course/unit handbook.

With careful preparation and a clear focus on the learning outcomes and assignment guidelines you can ensure that you are successful in your written assessments. Taking notice and acting on the feedback you receive will enable you to develop your academic writing style to be successful in your written assessments and meet the demands of a degree programme.

Chapter summary

This chapter has used student experiences to explore the processes that need to be undertaken in order to successfully complete a written assessment. It has emphasised the importance of good preparation that includes planning time for finding and reading relevant literature prior to beginning to write the assignment.

Developing a concise, academic writing style, writing critically, using feedback and avoiding plagiarism are the other elements that need to be considered if you are to gain a mark that reflects the efforts you have made.

Activities: brief outline answers

Activity 2.2: Critical thinking (page 17)

Below is a summary of the answers to the questions posed below.

What action might Jenny have taken to avoid failing her assignment?

*   Adequately prepare by ensuring that she has understood the assignment task, word allowance and the format in which it has to be submitted.
*   Create an assignment template.
*   Create an initial timeline.
*   Read the learning outcomes and ensure all the required content is included in a list of key words.
*   Attend any relevant study skills or library workshops.
*   Access core text and any recommended reading. Use key words to search for additional information.
*   Read and make notes so that she begins to understand the topic in depth and has paraphrased what she has read to avoid plagiarism.
*   Develop an assignment plan and detailed weekly timetable, identifying specific days on which work on the assignment will be undertaken.
*   Discuss assignment plan with module, course or unit leader.
*   Use an academic writing style in her assignment, supporting all statements with a reference.
*   Check that the first draft addresses all the learning outcomes.
*   Check referencing is in the correct format.
*   Submit on time using the full word allowance.

How will Jenny know what she has done wrong?

Feedback from the marker will tell Jenny what she has done wrong. This will include the need to:

*   include content to address learning outcome 1;
*   use essay not report format, so need to remove heading and bullet point lists;
*   write in a more academic style, using references correctly;
*   read more widely.

What action can Jenny take to ensure her resubmission is likely to be successful?

*   Email the marker and request an appointment so she fully understands what amendments she needs to make to her original assignment.
*   Read the assignment feedback and make a note of any areas of the feedback she does not understand.

- Create a detailed plan of when the work on assignment will be completed.
- Look at page 4 and make sure she understands that she has not written this section in an academic style.
- Access some of the core texts and other academic literature and plan time to read them.
- Make sure all statements are supported with a reference, and access the university referencing guide and use to correct reference list.
- Attend a meeting with the marker, taking with her a copy of her failed assignment, a copy of the assignment with the revisions she has made so far, the feedback and her list of areas of feedback she does not understand.

Activity 2.7: Critical thinking (page 26)

Rewritten example in the third person (impersonal tense):

> During a recent placement on a surgical ward one of the patients was given a diagnosis of breast cancer. As an inexperienced student it was difficult to know what to say to comfort and support her. Bach (2011) suggests that caring is invisible but experienced in the nurse–patient relationship. Caring involves *alleviating psychological distress* and *being humane* . . .

Further reading

Howatson-Jones, L (2010) *Reflective practice in nursing*. Exeter: Learning Matters.

This book provides some very useful guidance on the use of a range of models of reflection suitable for structuring the reflection process.

Hutchfield, K (2010) *Information skills for nursing students*. Exeter: Learning Matters.

This book is particularly useful for students who need to improve their writing and library skills.

Price, B and Harrington, A (2010) *Critical thinking and writing for nursing students*. Exeter: Learning Matters.

If you need to improve your critical thinking and writing skills, then this is the book for you.

Price, G and Maier, P (2007) *Effective study skills*. Harlow: Pearson Education Press.

This book has two useful chapters on improving your reading techniques and effective note taking.

Rose, J (2007) *The mature student's guide to writing*, 2nd edition. Basingstoke: Palgrave Macmillan.

This book has a useful chapter on sentence construction, paragraphing and punctuation for those who need to improve their fundamental writing skills.

Useful websites

www.palgrave.com/skills4study/index.asp

This site is provided by the publishers Palgrave Macmillan and offers a range of useful online study resources.

www.rcn.org.uk/development/library/elibrary

If you are a member of the Royal College of Nursing (RCN), you can access their e-library to expand your access to literature beyond your university library.

www.vtstutorials.co.uk/

The Virtual Training Suite site was developed by university tutors and librarians. This excellent site provides free online tutorials on how to use electronic databases for health and social care students.

Chapter 3
Succeeding in practice assessments

Kay Hutchfield

NMC Standards for Pre-registration Nursing Education

This chapter will address the following competencies:

Domain 1: Professional values

1. All nurses must practise with confidence according to *The code: Standards of conduct, performance and ethics for nurses and midwives* (NMC, 2008), and within other recognised ethical and legal frameworks. They must be able to recognise and address ethical challenges relating to people's choices and decision-making about their care, and act within the law to help them and their families and carers find acceptable solutions.

6. All nurses must understand the roles and responsibilities of other health and social care professionals, and seek to work with them collaboratively for the benefit of all who need care.

9. All nurses must appreciate the value of evidence in practice, be able to understand and appraise research, apply relevant theory and research findings to their work, and identify areas for further investigation.

Domain 2: Communication and interpersonal skills

3. All nurses must use the full range of communication methods, including verbal, non-verbal and written, to acquire, interpret and record their knowledge and understanding of people's needs. They must be aware of their own values and beliefs, and the impact this may have on their communication with others. They must take account of the many different ways in which people communicate and how these may be influenced by ill health, disability and other factors, and be able to recognise and respond effectively when a person finds it hard to communicate.

Domain 3: Nursing practice and decision-making

1. All nurses must use up-to-date knowledge and evidence to assess, plan, deliver and evaluate care, communicate findings, influence change and promote health and best practice. They must make person-centred, evidence-based judgements and decisions, in partnership with others involved in the care process, to ensure high quality care. They must be able to recognise when the complexity of clinical decisions requires specialist knowledge and expertise, and consult or refer accordingly.

Domain 4: Leadership, management and team working

3. All nurses must be able to identify priorities and manage time and resources effectively to ensure the quality of care is maintained or enhanced.

continued . . .

4. All nurses must be self-aware and recognise how their own values, principles and assumptions may affect their practice. They must maintain their own personal and professional development, learning from experience, through supervision, feedback, reflection and evaluation.

NMC Essential Skills Clusters

This chapter will address the following ESCs:

Cluster: Care, compassion and communication

1. As partners in the care process, people can trust a newly registered graduate nurse to provide collaborative care based on the highest standards, knowledge and competence.

By the first progression point:

i. Articulates the underpinning values of *The code: Standards of conduct, performance and ethics for nurses and midwives* (the code) (**NMC, 2008**).

By the second progression point:

vi. Forms appropriate and constructive professional relationships with families and other carers.

Chapter aims

By the end of this chapter you should be able to:

- make an effective plan for your placement learning;
- maximise your practice learning and ensure that your practice assessments are successful;
- understand the support that is available during your practice experience.

Introduction

This chapter will use a series of scenarios to consider some of the issues that may arise in practice that could impact on your practice assessment. It will challenge you to familiarise yourself with the competencies, standards and related essential skills clusters set by the NMC (2010b) and measured by your practice assessments, so that you can be proactive in planning your practice experience. It will also enable you to understand what the NMC expects from a nursing student in terms of professional behaviour.

Case study: Nicky (1)

Nicky is 26 and a single mum. She did quite well at school until she was 17 when she became pregnant and left before completing her A level studies. The relationship with her boyfriend lasted a year after their son Dan was born and by then she was pregnant with her second child. Nicky had worked part-time in a supermarket until she began her nursing programme and is approaching the end of her first year. Nicky is hoping that a career in children's nursing will turn her life around.

Nicky is currently on placement on a general children's ward where she has already had a successful placement earlier in the year; she feels quite confident about passing her practice assessment for the end of Year 1. However, there is a problem: because of issues with child care she has changed her shifts and is finding it difficult to fit in time to complete her formative assessment before she has a two-week Christmas break from placement. When her link tutor visits the ward she asks Nicky and her fellow student Amy if they have completed their formative assessments. Amy is quick to confirm that she has and then starts to talk animatedly about the experiences she has had during the previous week. Nicky just smiles and nods, giving the impression that she too has completed her practice assessment documentation; after all, she will have it done as soon as she comes back to the placement after Christmas.

What Nicky had not considered was that heavy snow would severely disrupt her placement after Christmas. Although she had a mentor each shift, her main mentor had severe difficulties getting to work and Nicky also had to change some shift times because of her own travel difficulties, providing limited opportunities for them to complete the formative assessment. As the end of the placement loomed, Nicky began to panic. The formative part of her assessment documentation was almost complete and only needed some sections initialled and signed, but she had none of the summative elements completed.

Activity 3.1 — Critical thinking

Take a few moments to consider what you might have done if you were Nicky.

Would you have acted differently?

Compare your thoughts with the ideas presented at the end of the chapter.

Some students find asking for help difficult, but mentors and link tutors are there to support and guide students, not to punish them. Asking for help when problems first arise is a good way of ensuring they do not develop into much more serious problems.

Case study: Nicky (2)

On the last day of her placement Nicky decided that she would approach the nurse who had been her mentor for her last placement on the ward. She had worked some shifts with her recently, and she hoped the nurse would complete the summative element of her practice assessment documentation. However, before she approached the

continued . . .

nurse she copied her mentor's initials in to all the formative sections so that they appeared complete, but she did not complete the signature section.

The nurse Nicky approached was an experienced mentor and was immediately surprised that Nicky's mentor had only initialled and not signed sections of the document as she knew her to be meticulous with student assessment forms. To Nicky's dismay the nurse said she could not complete the assessment documentation but would keep it on the ward to discuss with Nicky's mentor the following day.

The next morning the nurse and Nicky's mentor realised that the practice assessment document had been falsified and contacted the link tutor. The link tutor asked the nurse and mentor to complete incident statements and to retain the practice assessment document until she could collect it from them later that day.

The next day Nicky was called in to see her personal tutor who presented her with the reports and falsified practice assessment documentation. Nicky admitted that she had panicked and acknowledged that she was wrong to forge her mentor's initials. Nicky was informed that this was a very serious breach of professional behaviour that would have to be referred to the university 'Fitness to practice' panel. This panel would decide what the consequences of Nicky's action would be.

Nicky's personal tutor (Sarah) explained that the falsification of documentation is a serious issue and is not one that can be dealt with by the personal tutor or even the programme director. Sarah advised her that the situation would be dealt with under the university Fitness for Practice policy so that an objective consideration of the facts of the case could by made. Sarah provided Nicky with a copy of the policy and explained the Fitness for Practice process to her. She also advised Nicky to contact the student union for support and referred her to the university counselling service as she was obviously upset.

Activity 3.2   *Leadership and management*

Take a moment to think about Nicky's behaviour. Access your copy of the *Guidance for students* (NMC, 2011a) and identify where Nicky's behaviour might fall short of the expectations the NMC has of nursing students.

If you were on the 'Fitness to practice' panel, what action would you recommend be taken against Nicky and how would you justify this recommendation?

Compare your ideas with the answer at the end of the chapter.

Nicky's story highlights that it is not enough to be technically skilled at nursing procedures. The NMC, the legal system and the general public all expect nurses to behave with integrity both at work and at home. Nurses hold a position of trust in society, and if they are proven to be dishonest or untrustworthy, then their registration is immediately placed in jeopardy.

This chapter will now continue to explore practice assessment under four main headings: preparation, making a plan, maximising practice learning, and using feedback and support constructively to ensure that you understand what you are required to do to achieve successful practice assessment outcomes.

Preparation for practice

What preparation will my university provide?

You will be given a three-year plan of your programme, which will indicate when your practice placements will occur, and your student handbook should inform you of the nature of those placements (e.g. community/inpatient/specialist) and the practice assessment that you need to complete. Your university will also have made links between the learning outcomes for your academic work and your placement experiences. Understanding what learning you need to achieve in practice is essential for success in your practice assessment.

Your university will also provide you with information on the practice assessment documentation so that you are aware of when and what needs to be completed. This preparation may take the form of formal teaching, group work or directed study. Whichever format it takes, it is important that you complete this preparation in advance of your placement. If in doubt, seek clarification from your personal tutor. Do not rely on information passed on by other students as it may not be correct.

Some placements will provide you with an orientation pack in advance of starting your placement; this will provide you with the opportunity to complete more detailed planning. Others will have this information online, so make sure you access all the available information before you begin your placement.

What else do I need to do before I go on placement?

There are four additional things you need to do before you start your placement.

1. Make a note of the learning outcomes for the placement.
2. Read through the practice assessment document and familiarise yourself with the competencies and essential skills you are expected to achieve during this placement.
3. Identify some relevant literature and research to read before and during your placement that will enable you to have some initial understanding of the needs of the service users you will meet on your placement.
4. Look back on your previous practice assessment documentation and identify any areas that you need to improve.

Activity 3.3   *Critical thinking*

Identify your next placement and complete the activities in the two sections above.

Access your last completed practice assessment document and read the comments that you and your mentor have made regarding your practice. Were there any areas that needed improvement? If there are, make a note of these.

You are now in a position to move on to the next stage and make an initial plan for your practice learning.

As this activity is personal to you, there is no worked example at the end of the chapter.

Making a plan for your practice experience

In order to remain focused on a successful practice assessment you will be expected to develop a plan or learning contract for each placement that reflects the learning outcomes and competencies you are required to achieve for that placement. A learning contract should include the goals you aim to achieve, the resources/learning opportunities you will need to achieve them and the date by which they will be achieved. For each learning contract there will be a formative stage when you will review what you have achieved and use feedback from your mentor to amend your learning contract to ensure that you are successful in your summative assessment of practice. In order to examine this process more closely we will return to the scenario about Jenny, the first-year adult nursing student who failed her formative assessment of practice (Chapter 1, Activity 1.5). If you have not read Chapter 1 or completed Activity 1.5, it is important that you do so before commencing Activity 3.4.

Activity 3.4   *Decision-making*

We will assume that the discussions outlined in Activity 1.5 in Chapter 1 occurred during the tripartite meeting between Jenny, her mentor and the link tutor. Think about what changes Jenny's mentor will expect to see in Jenny's behaviour to ensure that she passes her summative assessment of practice. Use the learning contract below to identify the goals (competencies and NMC Essential Skills Cluster) and action Jenny will need to take and compare your ideas with the example at the end of the chapter.

Goals	What do I need to do to achieve my goal?	What resources/ learning opportunities will I need?	Date to be achieved by

Jenny feels she has learnt a lot from this placement. She has realised how important it is: to listen to negative as well as positive feedback from her mentor; to seek explanation of any negative feedback rather than dismiss it as unimportant; and to seek a way to address any shortfalls. Jenny's next placement is in the community, and she is keen not to repeat her previous mistakes. She is clear about the learning objectives she needs to achieve but wants to ensure she presents herself in a professional manner and as a team player so she does not repeat the problems she experienced on the elderly care ward.

Case study: Jenny

Jenny has contacted her community placement and discovered the journey to this placement is quite straightforward, so getting to work on time should not be a problem. Jenny will spend the first four weeks with a health visitor, and she met her to discuss her draft learning contract. She asked the health visitor what she expected from first-year students when they went out on placements.

The health visitor said that based on her previous experience with students she could sum up her expectations under three headings.

1. *Look and behave like a professional.*
2. *Show an interest and listen to the conversation between client and health visitor.*
3. *Be respectful and non-judgemental; remember that you are in someone's home.*

Jenny was surprised at these comments as she assumed that all students would automatically behave professionally, but she remembered her last mentor, and asked the mentor to explain what she meant.

Well, over the years I have mentored lots of nursing students and the vast majority have been great but some have caused me embarrassment in front of clients. For example, the way you dress is important. One student turned up looking as if she was going clubbing; she had a low-cut dress and short skirt. She was really upset when I suggested this was not appropriate dress for visiting clients in their home. Another student thought it OK to wear torn jeans. It's just not the way to dress for work.

The other big problem is mobile phones. Several students have started texting while in the client's homes. It is so rude and disrespectful. I expect students to turn off their mobile phones and attend to what the client and I are discussing, not text a friend or look aimlessly around the client's front room. Imagine you are talking to a new mum about concerns she has about her baby's development. She is not going to think her concerns are being taken seriously if the student is sitting in the corner texting.

The really good students help by playing with or distracting a toddler or young child so the mother can talk to me without interruption. They act sensitively to the situation. They have also bothered to do some reading before they come on placement, so I will let you have some literature on developmental assessment and post-natal depression that would be useful for you to read before you start here next week.

Activity 3.5 **Critical thinking**

What do you think Jenny will add to her learning contract that will reflect what she has learnt from this discussion with the health visitor? What action will she take to ensure she meets the expectations of the health visitor?

Compare your ideas with those listed at the end of the chapter.

When you write your learning contract, remember to use SMART objectives. Your goals should be Specific, Measurable, Achievable, Realistic and Timed. By using your learning outcomes, competency standards and essential skills cluster as the focus for your goals, you are likely to have a successful practice assessment.

As an example, let us look at one of Jenny's learning outcomes, competencies and essential skills cluster for her community placement.

Learning outcome

This placement should enable you to describe the role community nurses can play in health promotion, and discuss the challenges and advantages of lone working.

To achieve this learning outcome Jenny has looked at the plan for her eight-week community placement and developed some questions to ask the health visitor and district nurse about how they see their health promotion role. She has noted that there are also school nurses and an outreach sexual health worker in the same team, and plans to try to spend at least a day with these professionals to extend her understanding of the range of health promotion activities. Her goals for this part of her learning contract are outlined in Table 3.1.

Domain 1: Professional values

9. *All nurses must appreciate the value of evidence in practice, be able to understand and appraise research, apply relevant theory and research findings to their work, and identify areas for further investigation.*

This is one of the competencies Jenny has to demonstrate during this placement. Jenny has already accessed the recommended community care textbooks and has identified some areas she wants to explore. In her learning contract she has identified the chapters she wants to read and plans to take a textbook with her to work to make good use of any time when her mentor may be busy completing client records or making confidential communications. She has also read the two articles that the health visitor gave her and plans to learn more about post-natal depression and child protection in order to discuss these topics with the health visitor and so demonstrate her ability to meet this competence.

Goals	What do I need to do to achieve my goal?	What resources/ learning opportunities will I need?	Date to be achieved by
Be able to describe the health promotion role of the health visitor, district nurse, school nurse and sexual health nurse	• Ask each professional to describe how they see their role in health promotion and compare with the literature. • Request time with each group of professionals to observe them at work and make notes on my observations.	Access to contact numbers for school nurse and sexual health outreach nurse to arrange practice experience	• During first week of placement. • By end of 4-week placement.
Be able to discuss the advantages and disadvantages of lone working	• Ask each professional to identify what they see as the advantages and disadvantages of lone working • Access the trust lone working policy	Access to lone working policy	• During first week of placement. • By end of first week of placement.

Table 3.1: Jenny's learning contract goals

Essential Skills Cluster: Care, compassion and communication

1. *As partners in the care process, people can trust a newly registered graduate nurse to provide collaborative care based on the highest standards, knowledge and competence.*

By the first progression point:

1.1. *Articulates the underpinning values of* The code: Standards of conduct, performance and ethics for nurses and midwives *(the code) (NMC 2008).*

41

1.2.   Works within limitations of the role and recognises own level of competence.

1.3.   Promotes a professional image.

1.4.   Shows respect for others.

1.5.   Is able to engage with people and build caring professional relationships

This is one of the Essentials Skills Clusters that Jenny is required to complete during this placement. Jenny feels that her initial conversation with the health visitor has enabled her to clearly understand the professional image she is expected to present. She has decided to go to a discount clothes shop and buy a pair of smart black trousers and a cardigan which she can add to her current wardrobe to ensure she has appropriate clothes for placements where she is not required to wear her student uniform. She has also asked to spend one day a week at a Sure Start Centre so she can improve her listening skills with children and families in order to meet 1.5. With a well-designed learning contract Jenny feels confident that she will be successful on this practice placement.

Maximising practice learning

Having made appropriate preparation and constructed a draft learning contract to discuss with your mentor, you will be in a good position to make maximum use of the learning opportunities your placement has to offer and address the demands of your practice assessment.

During your placement you will work alongside your mentor assessing, planning and delivering care. Take opportunities to have elements of your assessment documentation completed and signed off as you achieve each competence so that it becomes a process of continuous assessment. This will make completing the assessment documentation a less arduous task for your mentor, and leave more time for discussion and reflection at the formative and summative points of the assessment process.

As a student you have supernumerary status. This means that you are not part of the staffing numbers for the ward, unit or team you are allocated to, but can be involved in direct patient care under the supervision of your mentor and commensurate with your stage on the course/ programme. However, supernumerary status also means that you can be released to be involved in a range of client-focused activities as long as they enable you to meet specific learning outcomes and are agreed with your mentor. For example, on her last placement Jenny accompanied one of the elderly patients to an eye clinic where he was diagnosed with glaucoma. She learnt about the symptoms, diagnosis and treatment of glaucoma, which was not on her learning contract but nevertheless a useful learning experience.

Following a patient's journey can include accompanying patients for investigations, surgery and consultations, and can provide insight into the whole patient experience and enhance your ability to empathise with the patient or client.

A positive practice experience is reliant not only on planning and implementing an effective learning contract, but also on a mentor who is supportive but also challenges you and tests your knowledge.

Case study: Mark

Mark is a second-year mental health student. His current placement is with a community mental health crisis intervention team. The placement is interesting, but Mark finds the unpredictability and intensity of the work stressful. His mentor seems to be extremely knowledgeable; he has discovered that Mark is not confident in drug calculations and needs to extend his knowledge of some of the drugs the team regularly uses. He has also tested Mark's understanding of the Mental Health Act and the concept of mental capacity and consent. Mark is worried that he is not going to pass his formative assessment on medication management, so he asks if he can speak to his mentor at the end of a shift.

His mentor is surprised that Mark feels he is not doing well. He agrees that Mark could improve on his knowledge of some medications and the speed at which he completes drug calculations but he feels that Mark has improved in the first three weeks of his placement and does not anticipate any problems with him successfully completing his practice assessment. In fact, he has been impressed with Mark's understanding of some of the ethical and legal aspects of mental health and his sensitive involvement in patient care.

The positive feedback from his mentor is a motivator for Mark. He makes sure that he practises his drug calculations every shift and makes a list of medications that he needs to look up and make notes on their mode of action, dosages and contraindications for future use.

From Mark's experience you can see that mentors have a responsibility to identify areas where a student needs to improve and test the extent of their knowledge. In this way they are able to judge how well students meet the NMC standards. However, in the busy context of the NHS, mentors may not always provide students with positive feedback, so if in doubt, it is always best to ask.

Once students enter their third year there is an expectation that they will begin to work more independently as their knowledge and competence increases and they move closer to registration. However, for some students this final step can be very challenging. Sign-off mentors are allocated to support students at this final stage of their programme. Sign-off mentors are experienced mentors who have been assessed as qualified to undertake students' final assessment of practice prior to a registration.

Case study: Lucy

Lucy is a third-year student on her final extended 12 weeks of practice. Her sign-off mentor, Karen, has been through her previous practice documentation. Comments from her mentors suggest that Lucy is a well-motivated student who delivers a good standard of care and works well in a team. However, she notices that the majority of Lucy's previous mentors have commented that at times Lucy appears shy, quiet or lacking in confidence. When checking Lucy's learning contract, Karen notes that Lucy has identified improving her confidence as one of her goals but that the actions she has identified to achieve this are vague and non-specific.

continued . . .

Based on her previous experience of third-year students, Karen is concerned that Lucy will need to improve her confidence if she is to pass her final practice assessment. When she meets Lucy to discuss her learning contract she raises her concerns and makes some suggestions on how she can amend her learning contract so that her goals and actions are more specific and focused at improving her confidence.

Creating a meaningful learning contract is essential if improvement is to be achieved. In Lucy's case she needs to identify the causes of her lack of confidence and take specific action to improve.

Activity 3.6 — *Critical thinking*

What actions or activities do you think would help improve Lucy's confidence?

Complete this section of the learning contract below and then compare your ideas with the one at the end of the chapter.

Goals	What do I need to do to achieve my goal?	What resources/ learning opportunities will I need?	Date to be achieved by
Feel more confident in practice			

By using Karen's experience Lucy can make a more effective learning contract that should enable her to successfully complete her final practice assessment. Without a reasonable level of self-confidence Lucy will not be able to adequately advocate for her patients and meet the expectations of the NMC.

Using feedback and support

We have seen how Jenny, Mark and Lucy have benefited from listening and utilising feedback from their mentors to improve their practice and pass their practice assessments. Mentors are central to your development as a nurse, and this is why the NMC stresses that students should spend at least 40 per cent of their practice time working with their mentor.

However, what happens if your mentorship does not measure up to expectations or, like Nicky, something unexpected happens to disrupt your mentorship? It does not have to be bad weather – it may be ill health, a bereavement or changes in rostering that have not taken students into account. Without continuity of mentorship you will have difficulty completing your assessment documentation, as a new mentor may feel they have not worked with you sufficiently to sign and comment on your practice assessment documentation. So what should you do?

The first person to approach is the nurse responsible for students on your placement. This may be a senior nurse, ward/unit manager, practice placement facilitator or education practice lead. They should be experienced at planning student supervision and should be able to manage the situation and arrange a suitable mentor for you. If this strategy does not work, there are two people who are the most important to contact as soon as you experience or anticipate problems with mentorship: your personal tutor and the link tutor. They are responsible for ensuring that the placement has sufficient mentors to support students and so will be in a position to seek a solution on your behalf.

If you have been off sick during a placement, you will be expected to make up the hours you have missed. When planning this with your mentor, make sure that your personal tutor is happy with your plan and that you will have continuity of mentorship during your 'make up' shifts.

Very occasionally a mentor fails to provide adequate supervision or guidance to a student. This can be a difficult situation for the student, but it is important that you act to safeguard your assessment. An initial approach to the mentor regarding your learning contract may be all that is needed. If this fails, then it is important that you discuss your problem with a senior member of the team in your practice placement and email your personal tutor and link tutor to inform them of your concerns. In such situations it is important that you keep a record of incidents of poor supervision or poor practice so that you can provide evidence of your concerns that are factual and not subjective/personal.

If your concerns relate to poor practice on the part of your mentor, then communicating your concerns becomes urgent, and you need to access your university's student whistle-blowing policy to ensure you follow the correct procedure.

Service user feedback

It is now common for service users to contribute to practice assessment. It is important that you are aware where this type of assessment and feedback will occur in your programme and how it will be organised. It is important to involve service users in all aspects of the nursing curriculum in order to develop practitioners who are sensitive to the needs of those who use the service they provide.

Try to ensure that service user comments are authentic and include some discussion of areas where you might improve.

Chapter summary

Practice assessments represent 50 per cent of assessments within all pre-registration nursing programmes and must be successfully completed if you are going to register as a nurse. This chapter has used scenarios to explore how you can best prepare for your placements and practice assessments. It has emphasised how good preparation will ensure you maximise your learning opportunities and meet the requirements of your practice assessments.

Activities: brief outline answers

Activity 3.1: Critical thinking (page 35)

I hope that you have said that you would have been honest.

Nicky could have contacted her link tutor or personal tutor when she realised she had difficulties working with her mentor and completing her practice assessment on time.

Nicky could have been honest when her link tutor when asked if she had completed her formative assessment and then the link tutor could have managed the situation.

When the bad weather exacerbated the problem, Nicky should have contacted her personal tutor and link tutor for help.

Activity 3.2: Leadership and management (page 36)

The statement below is the section of the NMC (2011a) *Guidance for students* that relates to Nicky.

Cheating or plagiarising
- Cheating in examinations, coursework, clinical assessment or record books.
- Forging a mentor or tutor's name or signature on clinical assessments or record books.
- Passing off other people's work as your own.

By forging her mentor's initials Nicky's integrity was brought into question. The outcome of the fitness for practice panel hearing was that Nicky should be required to leave the programme with immediate effect.

Activity 3.4: Decision-making (page 38)

Goals	What do I need to do to achieve my goal?	What resources/ learning opportunities will I need?	Date to be achieved by
Arrive at work on time for all remaining shifts.	Not late for any shifts.	Set my alarm 15 minutes earlier. No late nights before an early shift.	
Arrive on shift with pen and notepad.	Positive feedback from my mentor.	Buy a pack of black pens and two small pocket-sized notebooks.	Before next shift.
Pin my wristwatch to my uniform each shift and buy a fob watch asap.	Positive feedback from my mentor.	Ask parents to purchase as part of my birthday present.	Next week (22nd July).

Goals	What do I need to do to achieve my goal?	What resources/ learning opportunities will I need?	Date to be achieved by
Continue progress in the development of essential nursing skills.	Positive feedback from my mentor.	Find opportunities each shift to participate in essential nursing skills.	By summative assessment.

Activity 3.5: Critical thinking (page 40)

As a result of her discussion with the health visitor, Jenny might include the following in her learning contract.

- Find suitable clothes she can wear on her community placements.
- Plan time to do preparatory reading.
- Seek advance information about families that are being visited so that she can behave appropriately in the clients' home.

To meet the expectations of the health visitor, it is important that Jenny remembers to:

- switch off her mobile phone before entering the client's home;
- avoid being distracted from listening to the client by other things in the home environment;
- focus her attention on listening to the health visitor and client conversation so that she can discuss any queries with the health visitor after the visit;
- be useful if she can – for example, entertain or distract children so that the health visitor and parent can focus on the purpose of the visit.

Activity 3.6: Critical thinking (page 44)

Goals	What do I need to do to achieve my goal?	What resources/ learning opportunities will I need?	Date to be achieved by
Feel more confident in practice	Make a list of any conditions and treatments that I need to revise and spend one day week studying one/some of these.	Devise a study timetable.	During first week of placement.

Goals	What do I need to do to achieve my goal?	What resources/ learning opportunities will I need?	Date to be achieved by
	Hand over my patients at the end of shifts and gain feedback from my mentor.	Develop a structured handover sheet.	By end of second week of placement.
	Take opportunity to telephone doctors regarding patients in my care rather than asking my mentor to do it for me.	Use the SBAR (situation, background, assessment, recommendation) format to develop concise telephone communication.	By end of second week of placement.
	Make a list of any questions I need to ask the consultant/ registrar when they see my patients.	Make sure patient's and relatives' questions are included.	By week 3.
	Begin to make referrals under supervision.	Access trust policy guidance on referrals.	By week 4.
	Under minimal supervision of my mentor support a first placement student to deliver fundamental care to patients.	Develop a plan for teaching, taking basic observations	By week 6.
	Under minimal supervision of my mentor manage a section of the ward and delegate care to other nursing staff.	Watch how my mentor delegates care and discuss her decision-making with her.	By week 10.

Further reading

NMC (2011) *Guidance for students*. Available at: **www.nmc-uk.org/Students/Guidance-for-students/**.

You should be familiar with the content and principles of this document so that you are fully aware of the professional behaviours expected of you as a nursing student.

NMC (2010) Standards for pre-registration nursing education. Available at: **http://standards.nmc-uk.org/Pages/Welcome.aspx.**

In this document the most relevant aspects for you to be aware of are the generic and field competencies, which are in Section 2, and the essential skills clusters in the Annexe section.

Standing, M (2011) *Clinical judgement and decision-making for nursing students*. Exeter: Learning Matters.

This excellent book will guide you to a better understanding of the decision-making process in clinical practice and will assist you to challenge and improve your clinical judgement.

Useful website

www.institute.nhs.uk/quality_and_service_improvement_tools

This link will take you to more information on the NHS Institute of Innovation and Improvement SBAR tool. Take some time to look at other tools on this site that have been developed to improve practice in health care.

Chapter 4
Succeeding in written examinations
Mooi Standing

NMC Standards for Pre-registration Nursing Education

This chapter will address the following competencies:

Domain 3: Nursing practice and decision-making

2. All nurses must possess a broad knowledge of the structure and functions of the human body, and other relevant knowledge from the life, behavioural and social sciences as applied to health, ill health, disability, ageing and death. They must have an in-depth knowledge of common physical and mental health problems and treatments in their own field of practice, including co-morbidity and physiological and psychological vulnerability.

Domain 4: Leadership, management and team working

4. All nurses must be self-aware and recognise how their own values, principles and assumptions may affect their practice. They must maintain their own personal and professional development, learning from experience, through supervision, feedback, reflection and evaluation.

NMC Essential Skills Clusters

This chapter will address the following ESCs:

Cluster: Organisational aspects of care

17. People can trust the newly registered graduate nurse to work safely under pressure and maintain the safety of service users at all times.

Cluster: Medicines management

33. People can trust the newly registered graduate nurse to correctly and safely undertake medicines calculations.

Chapter aims

By the end of this chapter you should be able to:

- describe different types of written exams you may face as a nursing student;
- understand how questions test different levels of critical thinking;

- identify ways to improve your performance during written exams;
- plan a revision timetable to prepare for all types of written exams;
- access and practise answering a wide range of exam questions;
- consider the relevance of written exam skills to nursing practice.

Introduction

Case study: Karl's mistaken assumption

Karl is a second-year nursing student who is sitting a written exam. The last time he sat an exam he remembered feeling tired halfway through it, so this time he drank two cans of an energy drink to help him stay alert. After nearly an hour Karl had to go to the toilet so he put this hand up to get permission. He was shocked when the invigilator asked him if he wanted to wait as the exam would be over in 35 minutes' time. His previous exam lasted two hours and he had convinced himself that it would be the same this time (despite the duration being written on the exam paper and pointed out by the invigilator at the start). Karl was in a panic as he had not finished the question he was answering, still had one more to do, and could not do either without having a toilet break (which the invigilator allowed). Afterwards Karl had time only to finish the question he was writing and plan out his answer to the last question.

Karl just did enough to get a pass mark. He was annoyed because: a) he had made a silly mistake in assuming the exam would take the same time as the one he took before; b) 'scraping' a pass did not truly reflect how much he knew; c) it dented his chances of getting a 2:1 overall degree classification (his other results had been at that level). Karl vowed not to let himself down like this again and to carefully check exam details in future.

Like Karl, during your nursing programme you are likely to sit written exams. The case study highlights the stressful nature of sitting exams and how easy it is to make mistakes and not communicate what you know. After reading this chapter you will hopefully come away from exams without regrets (unlike Karl), knowing that you performed to the best of your ability. This chapter looks at why nursing programmes might include written exams and gives examples of different types of exams that you could possibly be faced with. It explores how the wording of exam questions can give clues about what the examiners might be looking for in your answers (regarding different levels of critical thinking ability). Another case study about what can go wrong if exam preparation is poor and how to put this right to avoid any further disappointment (e.g. organise revision timetable/practise answering exam questions) is described. Tips to improve your chances of success during the exam are given, including looking after yourself, respecting examination rules and getting your brain into gear. Special considerations for disadvantaged students are outlined. Advice is offered about how to 'pick yourself up' and succeed at the second attempt if you fail an exam. To round things off the relevance of written exams to your future career as a Registered Nurse is outlined.

Why do you have to sit written exams and what form do they take?

Before starting a nursing degree, most students will have sat formal written exams to get a national qualification (e.g. GCSE/A level) awarded by an examination board (e.g. AQA).

As other chapters in this book reveal, written exams are just one part of a wide range of assessments designed to measure nursing students' academic and professional abilities. In the United Kingdom, the Nursing and Midwifery Council (NMC) has passed responsibility for setting written exams (and other assessments) to individual universities and colleges. It means that nursing examination papers are not set by a national body (unlike in secondary education). Instead, each university sets their own written exams to assess nursing students' achievement of learning outcomes, which are derived from the relevant NMC standards.

To succeed in written exams you have to show what you know about the topic in question. This chapter invites you to have a go at various activities to help you to gain confidence and develop your skills in answering exam questions. Activity 4.1 gives you a gentle introduction to testing yourself in this respect by asking you to reflect on what has been said so far.

Activity 4.1   *Reflection/critical thinking*

This activity is for you to test your knowledge and understanding of what has been said above about written exams. It also illustrates one of the ways that exam questions can be structured, selecting an answer from alternative options given.

Which of the following statements best describes how nursing written examinations are set?

a) The NMC sets national nursing exams.
b) Universities set nursing exams without reference to NMC standards.
c) The NMC has nothing to do with nursing exams.
d) Universities set nursing exams with reference to NMC standards.

The correct answer and a supporting rationale can be found at the end of the chapter.

In tackling Activity 4.1 you were asked to recall information and show that you understood it, and in doing so you had a small taste of what it's like to have your knowledge tested. If you got the question right, you might feel more confident and ready to move on. If you got it wrong, you have an opportunity to find out why and to learn from the experience. If nobody gets the question right, it would suggest that the question and/or paragraph are confusing! So what, if anything, does this tell us about the nature and purpose of written examinations?

1. *Showing what we know:* sitting written exams provides feedback about how much we have learned, how well we communicate it, and what we still need to learn.
2. *Formal recognition of learning* (part of a summative assessment): passing the exam enables progression to the next level of learning, or to completion of the nursing programme.

3. *Quality of the programme*: exam results also give an indication of how well students' teaching and learning experiences have prepared them to achieve success in exams.

Exams challenge you to show what you know when answering the questions. Traditionally, a big element of the challenge is in not knowing what the questions are going to be. While this may still be the case a lot of the time, in some exams you might be told what the questions are going to be beforehand (so you can focus on researching your answers). Terms used to describe variations in the types of written exams you might face are summarised below:

Being told or not told what the exam questions will be –

Unseen You do not know what the questions will be until the examination day.
Seen You are told the questions in advance in order to plan your answers.

Style of questions –

Long answer	You may have around 45–60 minutes to write each answer.
Short answer	You may have just a couple of minutes to write each answer.
MCQs (multiple choice questions)	You are given alternative answers to select from.

Medium of answering questions –

Handwritten	You write responses to questions in an answer booklet.
Online/computer assisted	You type responses to questions on a computer keyboard (this medium is often used to test numeracy skills in calculating the correct dosage of drugs).

The similarities between written assignments (Chapter 2) and written exams are that they invite you to show what you know regarding relevant learning outcomes; they recognise your achievements and they give an indication of how good learning and teaching experiences are.

In other ways, written exams differ from written assignments.

1. Examination conditions have much more formal proceedings with an invigilator in attendance to ensure rules are enforced, e.g. no talking to other candidates.
2. Exams usually have time constraints of between one and three hours, which means you have to answer all the necessary questions within the permitted timeframe for the exam.
3. Exams test your ability to cope with pressure, i.e. being able to manage 1. and 2. in order to perform your best in answering the questions as effectively as possible.

When sitting a written exam you are therefore subject to more rigorous regulation, control, scrutiny, time constraints, and the added pressure this entails, than in written assignments. You are likely to be asked to sit at least one of the above types of written exams during your nursing degree so it makes sense to check out what to expect as it will help you prepare and increase your chances of success. Activity 4.2 invites you to find out more about this.

In order to be sure about how many and what type of written exams you may be required
to sit, you need to be well informed about your nursing programme's assessment strategy.
Take a moment to look at your programme handbook and/or assessment handbook and
see when you have to sit a written exam, what type of exam it is, and how long each exam
lasts.

As this information is specific to your own programme, no outline answer is provided.

Having had a brief look at why it is necessary to sit written exams, and their various types, we
will next explore how exam questions are worded in testing a range of knowledge and skills.

How do exam questions assess nursing knowledge and skills?

Nursing knowledge includes a wide range of applied physical science (e.g. pharmacological
treatments), applied social science (e.g. communication skills), evidence-based research (e.g.
reducing infection rates), and reflective practice (e.g. learning from clinical experience). Nursing
knowledge is not static; it is developing all the time so you need to continually update what you
know. More importantly, you need to develop your critical thinking skills to review the adequacy
of your knowledge, build upon it, and apply theory to practice to benefit patients.

Nursing exam questions are therefore worded differently according to the level of critical thinking
they seek to elicit from candidates. Table 4.1 illustrates this by specifying six levels of critical
thinking (adapted from Bloom, 1956), identifying typical words used in questions associated with
probing each level of critical thinking, and showing how this relates to an everyday activity for
many nurses regarding the monitoring of patient blood pressure (BP).

Table 4.1 illustrates how being knowledgeable (knowing normal BP) is a starting point from which
you can:

- dig deeper for greater understanding (what this tells you about how the heart works);
- show how it informs your clinical activities (using devices to monitor BP);
- assess your patient's health and well-being (detect possible abnormalities in BP);
- take appropriate action in response to observational evidence (increase BP monitoring/refer
  to medical team);
- review the effectiveness of your actions (importance of accurate BP monitoring).

Activity 4.3 asks you to think of your own example of a nurse using different levels of critical
thinking.

Level of critical thinking assessed	Wording of questions to assess different levels	Example answer re nurse monitoring a patient's BP
Knowledge (remember)	define, describe, identify, list, state, outline	Adults normal resting BP is 120 (systolic) over 80 (diastolic).
Comprehension (understand)	explain, summarise, interpret, paraphrase, discuss	Systolic is when heart contracts so BP is higher than diastolic when it refills.
Application (practice)	apply, show, demonstrate, illustrate, give example of	Sphygmomanometers are used by nurses to monitor patients' BP.
Analysis (examine)	examine, compare, contrast, explore, assess	If a patient's BP is too high or too low, there may be a health problem.
Synthesis (transform)	develop, plan, create, propose, compile, integrate	Step up BP and other observations and refer patient to medical team.
Evaluation (critique)	evaluate, critique, appraise, justify, conclude	BP monitoring is vital to assess health of a patient's heart/circulation.

Table 4.1: Examining different levels of nurses' critical thinking in monitoring BP

Activity 4.3   *Critical thinking*

This activity is intended to help you to explore the difference between the levels of critical thinking identified above. The first two columns of the table below are the same as in Table 4.1, but the third column has been left blank. This is for you to fill in. Choose your own example of a nursing activity, identify knowledge you think is needed to perform it, and then work through the other five levels of critical thinking in relation to your example. In doing so, you will get a taste of how to respond to the different levels of questioning in written exams.

As this activity is for you to self-assess your understanding of the different levels of critical thinking in relation to your own example of a nursing activity, no outline answer is provided. You might find it interesting to do peer assessment by comparing your example/responses with a colleague because different points of view can help to clarify and reinforce learning.

continued . . .

Level of critical thinking assessed	Wording of questions to assess different levels	Example answer
Knowledge (remember)	define, describe, identify, list, state, outline	
Comprehension (understand)	explain, summarise, interpret, paraphrase, discuss	
Application (practice)	apply, show, demonstrate, illustrate, give example of	
Analysis (examine)	examine, compare, contrast, explore, assess	
Synthesis (transform)	develop, plan, create, propose, compile, integrate	
Evaluation (critique)	evaluate, critique, appraise, justify, conclude	

In looking at how written exam questions test a wide range of nursing knowledge, it was noted that they also test critical thinking skills. This is important as graduate nurses need to be effective critical thinkers (Price and Harrington, 2010) in anticipating and responding intelligently to patients' health problems (as well as being practically and interpersonally competent). As you progress from novice student to registered nurse you will be asked to demonstrate greater levels of critical thinking regarding the theory and practice of nursing. For example, by the first progression point you will be expected to have gained certain knowledge and understanding. By the second progression point you will be expected to apply theory to inform the care of patients and the assessment of their health needs. By completion of the nursing programme you will need to apply all six levels of critical thinking, including synthesis (e.g. ability to plan) and evaluation of care. While written exams cannot test clinical nursing skills, they can test the different levels of critical thinking needed to inform sound, evidence-based nursing. You may, therefore, be asked to sit a written exam at one or more significant milestones during your nursing programme.

In exploring the link between critical thinking and the wording of questions that assess each level (Table 4.1 and Activity 4.3) you can begin to anticipate what examiners are searching for in your answers. However, you need to do more to increase your chances of success, so we will now look at what you should do to fully prepare for a written exam.

What is the best way to prepare for a written exam?

In a way, sitting a written exam is like having a photograph taken because it provides a snapshot of what you know at a specific moment in time. Very few people are naturally photogenic, always looking good even when they are not expecting their picture to be taken. Similarly, very few people find succeeding in written exams effortless; most of us have to work hard at revision if we are to do well. Just as posing for a formal portrait photograph can make you self-conscious and not look your best, the prospect of sitting a written exam can make you feel anxious, which may result in you not performing to the best of your ability. The following case study illustrates how a student learnt to break the cycle of getting very anxious about exams, putting off preparing for them, and getting disappointing results.

> ### Case study: Learning the value of good preparation the hard way
>
> *Michelle, age 21, is a third-year nursing degree student. When Michelle was at secondary school she was very nervous about exams. Her reaction ranged from complete denial (block out all thought of exams) to total saturation (spend all day and night before an exam 'cramming'). When Michelle sat her A levels she was tired from lack of sleep, struggled to concentrate, and got confused about some of the facts she was trying to recall. Instead of getting the three Bs predicted she got C/C/D. She was angry for not doing herself justice and not getting the grades for her preferred university. Michelle got a job in a department store for a year while studying independently to resit exams. She was disciplined and focused, revising subjects a couple of hours every other evening, and got hold of past exam questions to practise doing timed answers. When Michelle resat her A levels, her grades went up to A/B/C and she got a place at her first-choice university. Michelle has passed all of her nursing degree assessments so far, including two written exams that she made sure she began revising for well in advance.*

Michelle's story shows how fear of exams and lack of confidence is self-fulfilling unless you channel your nervous energy into positive action to plan and execute a revision strategy. How you revise is largely a matter of personal choice, so the onus is on you to organise it. This can be quite challenging because if you are very nervous about exams (like Michelle) it can muddle your thinking and make you forgetful and disorganised. The following common-sense principles can be applied to guide the organisation of your individual revision plans:

Get organised

- Plan ahead. See when next written exam is due from your programme handbook.
- Find out what type of written examination it will be, e.g. seen, unseen, MCQ, online.
- Identify learning outcomes assessed at first and second progression points or registration.

- Revise notes (lecture/seminar/independent study) regarding topics to be assessed.
- Don't be intimidated by exams because if you prepare well, you will most likely pass.
- Don't put off revision until the last minute, creating information overload, stress and panic.
- Don't do exhausting all-day marathon revision sessions. One to two hours a day is better.

As Michelle discovered (the hard way), good preparation is the best way to overcome anxieties about exams. The starting point in getting organised is to know when, where and what type of written exam you have to sit (as you were asked to do in Activity 4.2). This enables you to plot a timeline of revision sessions in the weeks leading up to a written exam (as planned in Chapter 2 regarding written assignment deadlines, on page 23). Unlike lecture timetables, which are organised by the university, revision timetables are mainly your own responsibility to plan and implement. Taking control of your own exam revision in this way can help you to feel more positive and less like a victim of circumstance. You can then check what topics you need to know about, and set about revising those for five to ten hours a week, the month before an exam.

Activity 4.4 *Time management*

If you are to benefit from reading this chapter it will be because it has nudged you to take more control of your fate by setting time aside to prepare properly for written exams, and thereby increase your chances of success. This activity is designed with that in mind.

1. Decide what format you wish to use to create your own revision timetable: for example, electronic format (e.g. schedule function on laptop or mobile phone, Word or Excel document) or handwritten (e.g. calendar, diary, filoFAX®, wall chart).
2. Input/write down the title and type (unseen, seen, MCQ, online) of your next written exam on the date and time in question and make a note of its duration.
3. Make a note-to-self to 'start revision' on the Sunday/Monday of the fourth week before the exam, and allocate five to ten hours each week leading up to it. Schedule one to two hours a day for five days each week (so you get revision-free days) or two to three hours every other day. If you do not yet have details of other commitments, e.g. shifts, during the revision period, be prepared to swap times around when you have them.
4. Identify the learning outcomes being assessed from the student/programme/module handbook and assessment guidelines. Summarise and/or cross-reference these (document, page, item number) in your revision timetable to guide what you revise.
5. Identify topics to revise (from the learning outcomes, module contents, notes from lectures/seminars/independent study etc., books, articles and online resources) and allocate slots in your revision timetable to read up on/make notes about each topic. Build in time at the end for an overview of everything you revised so that you don't forget what you revised earlier, and to help you integrate what you have learned.

As this activity is an exercise in your own time management, no outline answer is provided at the end of the chapter.

Revising relevant material thoroughly in readiness to have your knowledge tested is vital, but written exams do not simply test subject knowledge and critical thinking skills. They also test your skills in the process of sitting exams, such as keeping cool under pressure, focusing on what questions ask, and being organised in your answers. For example, you might be well informed about a subject, but if you misread a question or you are unclear what it is asking for, you will be unable to communicate what you know in a time-constrained written exam. So, in addition to revising nursing studies, you also need to be familiar with the format of exam papers and adept at knowing what the questions are asking for. The best way to do this is to gain experience in answering exam questions, because skills needed to succeed in written exams are learned and improved through practice, as the following tips suggest.

Get practising

- Include practising exam questions within your revision timetable (see Activity 4.4).
- Find examples of questions from past exam papers (e.g. tutor, library archive, online).
- Devise your own questions regarding the learning outcomes that are being assessed.
- Study questions individually/with others to quiz each other about key points to include.
- Practise answering questions in the time you will have during the exam.
- Review answers individually/with others; identify and learn from mistakes/omissions.
- Find out date of mock exam and make sure you attend to practise in exam conditions.

The next activity gives you a helping hand in finding relevant ready-made tests of nursing knowledge and the chance to practise a broad range of short answer questions and MCQs.

Activity 4.5   *Critical thinking and decision-making*

This activity directs you to websites to practise testing what you know about calculating drug doses and different aspects of nursing. You will need internet access for at least one hour.

1. This will give you experience of an online quiz to test your drug calculation skills. Go to www.testandcalc.com/quiz/index.asp – you will see links to four 20-item quizzes (metric conversions, fluid dosage, tablet dosage, IV drop rate calculations). Each quiz has a help button you can click if you need a bit more guidance. Click on whichever quiz you wish to attempt, read the instructions, click 'Begin test', and input your answers to the questions. You can click 'check' (left of screen under each question) to see if you are right. You can also click 'show me the correct answer' or 'show me the solution', i.e. how to work out correct answer (right of both screen and question). Some of the questions may seem quite simple, but be wary, because if you switch off concentration, you could make an error. If you find that you have made mistakes, wait for about a week, then repeat the quiz to see if you have learned how to get every question right. Attempt the other three calculation quizzes when you are ready to.

continued . . .

2. This will give you experience of MCQ exams testing nursing knowledge, critical thinking and decision-making. Go to www.nclexonline.com – click 'Click here to register' and opt for standard (free) membership. Follow the instructions so that you can log in to the website. You will now have access to the MCQ exams – click 'NCLEX EXAM' on the toolbar at the top of the screen – then scroll down to the bottom half of the page to 'NCLEX Practice test' section – click on one of the practice tests and select an answer to each of the questions (25–30 in total, usually). When you have finished the last question you will get your test score. You will also have access to the answer guide and rationale used to determine what was correct or incorrect. Don't forget to log out. You can log back in again at any time to attempt other MCQs and/or have repeat attempts to see if you can improve your scores.

Both websites in this activity have answer guides to questions and explanations that you can check. As a registered member of nclexonline.com you can also post feedback, point out any typographical errors you might find, and raise queries about the questions or the answer guides.

As this activity is for your own practice using the internet, no outline answer is provided at the end of the chapter.

Having invested your time wisely in revising for and practising exams you will be much better prepared to perform to the best of your ability on the day of the exam itself.

Tips to improve your chances of success during written exams

Sitting exams can be a bit nerve-racking, and feeling anxious about it is quite natural. Anxiety is helpful if it makes you more alert and attentive but is unhelpful if it stops you doing your best. This section looks at how to look after yourself, respect examination rules, and get your brain into gear on the day of the exam so that you can show what you know to the best of your ability.

Look after yourself

Taking exams can be stressful, so you need to 'nurse' yourself to help ensure that you are as physically fit and mentally sharp as you can be. With this in mind it is best to avoid drinking alcohol for a few days before an exam. Treat yourself to some of your favourite meals in the week leading up to the exam to help stimulate your appetite, ensure you are well nourished, and provide a pleasant distraction from studying. Exercise can help to work off the calories, relieve any nervous tension, and boost respiration/circulation/oxygenation. Try to have a good night's sleep before an exam, and carbohydrates for breakfast to boost energy levels. Make sure that you have a foolproof plan for waking up on time, and getting to the exam centre 10–15 minutes early so you can breathe a little easier and gather your thoughts.

Respect examination rules

Make sure you have read and understood examination regulations and procedures, and that you adhere to them to avoid disadvantaging yourself and other candidates. Your university's examination procedures will tell you about identity checks/candidate numbers, what you are allowed and not allowed to take into the exam with you, the rule of silence in the examination room, penalties for cheating, the role of the invigilators and examination officers, and what to do if you have a query or need more paper.

Get your brain into gear

Once you are given permission to start the exam it is down to you to show what you know. In order to do yourself justice and perform well under examination conditions, you need to manage time well and pay attention to details.

Manage time well
- Be aware of how long the exam lasts.
- Take a couple of minutes at the beginning to familiarise yourself with the format and questions.
- Leave five to ten minutes at the end to check your answers and fill in any gaps.
- Estimate how much time to spend on each question (divide remaining time by the number of questions to answer).
- Check time occasionally during the exam to keep on track in answering the questions.
- If you get stuck, don't waste time; move on to other questions to earn more marks. It may help to clear the 'thought block', enabling you to go back to a problem question.

Pay attention to details
- Be absolutely clear what the exam requires you to do as any lapse in concentration could be costly.
- Read through the exam paper to see what the questions are.
- Check instructions so you know whether you have to attempt all questions or if you have a choice.
- If there are different sections, answer the right number/type of questions from each section.
- Read questions carefully to answer only what is asked. Don't 'go off on a tangent' – you won't get marks for irrelevant material.
- Make it clear which questions you are answering.
- Write legibly.
- Note whether marks for questions/parts of questions vary and weight answers accordingly (spend more time on high-value questions).
- Make sure that you have written your candidate number on the answer booklet and on any extra paper (or computer screen page for online tests).

Special considerations for disadvantaged students

Most universities have policies and procedures whereby special arrangements can be put in place to enable students with disabilities to sit written exams. This might include giving more time to a dyslexic student to complete an exam, or arranging for a scribe to write out answers dictated by a student who has lost the use of an arm due to injury or disease. It is usually the student's responsibility to give notice requesting such considerations from the university well before the exam is due. Evidence from a chartered educational psychologist regarding dyslexia or a medical consultant regarding physical disability may be required to support a student's application for special considerations.

What to do if you fail

If the worst happens and you fail a written exam, you have the right to appeal, as laid out in your university's appeals procedure. This would not usually allow the judgement of the examiners in marking your paper to be questioned. If you have reason to believe there were irregularities in how the exam was conducted or there were special circumstances affecting your performance on the day, then you could ask for this to be taken into consideration. If the appeal fails and you have a chance to resit the exam, you need to take note of the following.

- Remember that a 'fail' is a judgement on your exam performance *not* you as a person.
- Find out why you did not pass from written feedback and by speaking to your tutor.
- Identify if it was because you lacked knowledge or the ability to put it down on paper.
- Agree an action plan with your tutor to address deficits in knowledge or exam technique.
- Implement the action plan (e.g. improve study skills, revise knowledge, practise exams).
- Learn from this experience to maximise your chances of passing at the second attempt.

Are skills in passing written exams transferable to practising as a nurse?

If the summative assessments in your nursing programme include written exams, you will not be able to qualify as a registered nurse unless you pass them. Beyond this, what use are they? Nurses have been described as *knowledgeable doers* (Benner, 1984) because good nursing care is underpinned by sound professional knowledge. Written exams are one way of prompting nursing students to 'show what they know' in this respect. Public confidence in nurses might be boosted by knowing that they have had to pass written and practical exams. Whenever you care for a patient the adequacy of your knowledge and skills are tested as you have to be able to explain/justify/defend every clinical decision/nursing action you take. You need good writing skills to record the care that you give patients, and these care records are subject to ongoing clinical audit. You may also be called upon to write witness statements in investigations into the quality of care or professional conduct. Hence, written exams give you an opportunity to practise critical thinking and writing skills that graduate nurses need to use in high-pressure nursing contexts throughout their working lives. You will have further opportunities, through continuing professional development (CPD), to reflect, explore and develop these critical thinking skills throughout your nursing career.

Chapter summary

This chapter has: described the different types of written exams you might be asked to sit (knowledge); discussed the purpose of written exams (understanding); engaged you in activities to sharpen up your skills in revising for and sitting exams (application); explored the factors that prevent effective preparation for exams, such as feeling nervous or being disorganised (analysis); developed strategies such as organising a revision timetable, practising exam questions, and managing time effectively to overcome difficulties (synthesis); and reviewed the relevance of skills to pass written exams to nursing practice (evaluation). In doing so, it has demonstrated how to address all the different levels of critical thinking skills (adapted from Bloom, 1956) that graduate nurses need to use in delivering high-quality care.

Activities: brief outline answers

Activity 4.1: Reflection/critical thinking (page 52)

The correct answer is d). Options a), b) and c) are wrong.

a) NMC sets national standards not exams.
b) Universities do set exams but saying they don't refer to NMC standards is untrue.
c) It is untrue that NMC has nothing to do with it as NMC standards influence exams.

Further reading

Cottrell, S (2012) *Exam skills handbook: achieving peak performance.* Basingstoke: Palgrave Macmillan.

The latest edition of this practical book helps students to do their best in exams.

Starkings, S and Krause, L (2010) *Passing calculations tests for nursing students.* Exeter: Learning Matters.

A very helpful step-by-step guide in how to calculate drug doses accurately and pass nursing calculations tests.

Useful website

www.authenticworld.co.uk

This website offers online interactive learning/assessment in how to reduce errors in the administration of medicines to enhance patient safety. Many universities have bought a licence to use this website, and if yours is one of them, you can freely access the resources.

Chapter 5
Succeeding in portfolios

Kay Hutchfield

NMC Standards for Pre-registration Nursing Education

This chapter will address the following competencies:

Domain 1: Professional values

9. All nurses must appreciate the value of evidence in practice, be able to understand and appraise research, apply relevant theory and research findings to their work, and identify areas for further investigation.

Domain 2: Communication and interpersonal skills

7. All nurses must maintain accurate, clear and complete records, including the use of electronic formats, using appropriate and plain language.

Domain 3: Nursing practice and decision-making

10. All nurses must evaluate their care to improve clinical decision-making, quality and outcomes, using a range of methods, amending the plan of care, where necessary, and communicating changes to others.

Domain 4: Leadership, management and team working

4. All nurses must be self-aware and recognise how their own values, principles and assumptions may affect their practice. They must maintain their own personal and professional development, learning from experience, through supervision, feedback, reflection and evaluation.

NMC Essential Skills Clusters

This chapter will address the following ESCs:

Cluster: Care, compassion and communication

5. People can trust a newly qualified graduate nurse to engage with them in a warm, sensitive and compassionate way.

By the first progression point:

v. Evaluates ways in which own interactions affect relationships to ensure that they do not impact inappropriately on others.

By entry to the register:

xiii. Through reflection and evaluation demonstrates commitment to personal and professional development and life-long learning.

continued . . .

Cluster: Organisational aspects of care

12. People can trust the newly registered graduate nurse to respond to their feedback and a wide range of other sources to learn, develop and improve services.

By the second progression point:

iii. Uses supervision and other forms of reflective learning to make effective use of feedback.

By entry to the register:

vi. Actively responds to feedback.

14. People can trust the newly registered graduate nurse to be an autonomous and confident member of the multi-disciplinary or multi-agency team and to inspire confidence in others.

By the first progression point:

iv. Reflects on own practice and discusses issues with other members of the team to enhance learning.

Chapter aims

By the end of this chapter you should be able to:

* demonstrate awareness of the range of portfolio styles;
* identify the core principles of successful portfolio development;
* implement the principles of maintaining a professional profile (portfolio).

Introduction

As portfolios can take many forms depending on the learning outcomes that have to be achieved, the focus of this chapter will be on effectively using the principles of successful portfolio development. The chapter will explore the nature of portfolios and how to complete a variety of formative and summative portfolio assessments. It will identify the most common forms of portfolios used in nurse education programmes and required by the NMC to demonstrate continuing personal professional development, and it is designed to complement another book in this series, *Success with your professional portfolio for nursing students* (Reed, 2011).

What is a portfolio?

The word 'portfolio' literally means a case for carrying papers, but today the term is generally used to describe a collection of evidence that might refer to an individual's art work, financial assets or roles and responsibilities, for example. In the context of nursing, the term is used to describe a collection of evidence that demonstrates knowledge, skills and experiences acquired to meet the demands of nursing education and professional practice. They may take the form of manual or electronic records.

In university you may be required to provide a variety of portfolios in order to meet the assessment needs of your nursing programme. However, maintaining a professional portfolio will extend beyond your student studies in to your professional life, as the NMC requires all registered nurses to maintain a portfolio in the form of a *personal professional profile*, as outlined in *The prep handbook* (NMC, 2011b).

This chapter will consider developing successful portfolios under three headings.

- Portfolio as a 'snapshot' of specific knowledge and skills.
- Portfolio as a process of reflection and development.
- Portfolio as a record of achievement.

Portfolio as a 'snapshot' of specific knowledge and skills

As part of your programme you may be required to produce a portfolio that provides evidence of your ability to meet specific criteria.

Case study: Amy

Amy has just started the second year of her nursing programme. One of her assessments for this year is a portfolio that demonstrates her ability to meet the criteria for progression to Year 3.

The criteria require Amy to demonstrate her ability to:

- work more independently, with less direct supervision, in a safe and increasingly confident manner;
- demonstrate potential to work autonomously, making the most of opportunities to extend knowledge, skills and practice.

Amy is very concerned about her ability to meet these criteria as she is not very confident in clinical practice and some of her mentors have commented that she needs to be more assertive in her communication with other professionals.

Here we can see that Amy has to meet very specific outcomes if she is going to progress to the third year of her nursing programme. She will need to produce a successful portfolio to achieve this.

Activity 5.1   *Critical thinking*

The guidelines for Amy's portfolio state that her portfolio should have three sections. The first section needs to demonstrate how she has planned to meet the criteria. The second section must include evidence that the criteria have been met, and the third section has to be a reflection on her progress on meeting the criteria and an action plan for further development in Year 3.

Given Amy's lack of confidence, what would you include in her plan to make this section of her portfolio successful?

Compare your thoughts with those at the end of the chapter.

Using the portfolio guidelines effectively is essential if you are going to develop a successful portfolio. In this situation it is important that Amy makes an effective plan and then reviews and revises it as outcomes are achieved.

When developing an effective personal/professional development plan it is important to begin with an evaluation of your current situation so that your strengths as well as your weaknesses are considered. This normally takes the form of a SWOT analysis. Table 5.1 is an example of what Amy's SWOT might look like.

Strengths	*Weaknesses*
– Good knowledge of altered physiology and basic pharmacology.	– My shyness impacts on my ability to effectively advocate for patients.
– Confident with drug calculations.	– My shyness can be interpreted as a lack of confidence and enthusiasm.
– Good academic marks.	– I often avoid taking the lead or making suggestions for patient care.
– Kind and thoughtful.	
– Conscientious and hardworking.	– I tend always to ask for direction from my mentor for patient care.
– Not over-confident.	– I do not like phoning/speaking to doctors.
	– Because of my shyness I do not always seek learning opportunities that are available.

Table 5.1: Amy's SWOT analysis

Opportunities	*Threats*
– Two five-week placements coming up where I can practise developing my communication with colleagues. – Second five-week placement is in the community where I can begin to improve my ability to work safely with less direct supervision. – Specialist nurses work within both placement areas and I need to make sure I access these learning opportunities.	– I allow my shyness to impact on my need to improve my assertive communication skills. – I do not make my needs clear to my mentor.

Table 5.1: Continued

From her SWOT analysis Amy is able to extract goals for her personal development plan. Table 5.2 is an example of two goals that Amy might set herself.

When creating her development plan Amy used SMART objectives (Specific, Measurable, Achievable, Realistic and Timed). By using this approach, this section of her portfolio is likely to be successful as she will have created a plan that is specific, is achievable and can be measured and evaluated.

If you want further information about the SBAR (situation, background, assessment, recommendation) communication system, SMART objectives and personal development planning, please refer to another book in this series, *Information skills for nursing students* (Hutchfield, 2010).

To be successful in the second section of her portfolio, Amy must include evidence that the criteria have been met. She will have presented her development plan as part of her learning contract for each placement. This will be agreed with her mentor and will be part of her evidence. Amy will use her mentor's written comments in her assessment documentation as evidence of achieving the competencies needed to progress to Year 3. Using both her placements will provide her with the time she needs to develop her communication skills and independence in practice.

Amy will ensure that she completes the student section of her assessment of practice documentation before her formative and summative interviews with her mentor. This way she can identify where she feels she has developed, as well as situations where she still needs to improve. This type of preparation prior to meetings with her mentors is likely to result in a balanced and productive discussion where her mentors' and Amy's perceptions of her progress can be explored. This activity will add to the quality of the evidence she will be able to include in her portfolio and increase the chances of this section of the portfolio being successful.

For the third section of the portfolio Amy has to write a reflection on her progress on meeting the criteria and an action plan for further development in Year 3 as she progresses to registration.

Specific objective	How will I know when this is achieved?	What resources will I need?	When will this be achieved by?
1. Improve my communication skills by using the SBAR tool for communicating with my mentor and medical staff.	When I no longer feel uncomfortable communicating my views on my patients' condition or needs to my mentor or other health and social care professionals. When feedback from my mentor confirms that I appear more confident when communicating.	A copy of the SBAR tool to take to placements as a reference. Encouragement from my mentor for me to take every opportunity to hand over my patients to colleagues at the end of each shift.	Review progress after three weeks. Revise plan if needed. Achieved by end of first five-week placement.
2. Require less direction when caring for patients with simple health needs.	When I can evaluate care and make sound recommendations for changes in my patients' care plans. When I consistently deliver safe care with minimal input from my mentor.	Encouragement from my mentor for me to make judgements about patient need and discuss with her rather than ask for direction.	Improved by end of first five-week placement. Achieved fully during second five-week placement.

Table 5.2: Part of Amy's development plan

The key to an effective reflection is to keep a record of the journey you have taken so that you can return to the thoughts and feelings you were experiencing at certain times. This record should always include any critical incidents that mark a turning point in your development. This does not have to be a life-or-death situation but one that has a significant impact on your development.

Amy has decided to make a record of her journey in a journal that focuses just on the progression aspect of her development. When she completed her research on SBAR and assertiveness she wrote about how she felt and the self-doubt she experienced. She also wrote about her experiences practising using the SBAR tool and being more assertive in her everyday life. On placements, Amy tried to make a note in her journal each day as this allowed her to record how well she was implementing her plan, how effective it was in increasing her confidence and independence, and the challenges she faced.

Case study: Critical incident

Amy was on shift with her mentor. At hand-over Amy was interested in one particular patient who had been admitted with keto-acidosis. She had never cared for a person with diabetes before although she had a good theoretical understanding of the condition. She was disappointed when the patient was not allocated to her mentor. The unit was busy, and Amy realised that if she did not assert herself she would once again miss a learning opportunity. She used the SBAR format when she spoke to her mentor and negotiated to spend the second half of the shift working with the nurse caring for the diabetic patient. She was also surprised when her mentor suggested that Amy arrange to spend an afternoon with the diabetic nurse in her clinic to gain a greater insight into the management of the condition in the community.

When Amy came to record the incident in her journal she remembered how nervous she had felt when she had spoken to her mentor about her learning needs. Normally, she would have said nothing and missed the learning opportunity. When she thought about why she had behaved differently in the past, she realised that she anticipated a negative response to her request. Her experience had been the exact opposite. Her mentor had been willing to negotiate and also expand Amy's learning opportunities. She seemed pleased at Amy showing an interest. From this incident Amy learnt that making her own learning needs known was important and that such requests were likely to be received positively.

Amy wrote this incident up as a critical incident to include as evidence of her development for her portfolio.

When Amy comes to write her reflection she will be able to read her journal and extract key factors that influenced her progress and thereby add analysis to her reflection. It will include other critical incidents and a description of what she has learnt about herself as a result of her reflections to demonstrate her increasing self-awareness. The ability to reflect critically will be essential for success in this section of the portfolio.

To extend your knowledge of the process of reflection, please access another book in the series, *Reflective practice in nursing* (Howatson-Jones, 2010).

Portfolio as a process of reflection and development

The introduction of electronic or e-portfolios has made portfolio a more dynamic process that enables students to share more easily their portfolios with others (e.g. their personal tutor) and participate in discussions without the necessity of a face-to-face meeting. Although paper portfolios still enable you to record critical incidents and receive feedback, an electronic portfolio enables you more easily to extract relevant content from your reflective journal for inclusion in your reflective assignments. Some students may also prefer to keep an online rather than a paper journal for privacy reasons.

Rather than a static snapshot or collection of evidence an e-portfolio can become a record of the processes that have enabled a student to complete the journey to registration. It is highly likely that you will be required to keep such a portfolio as part of your programme.

The inclusion of critical or pivotal incidents in e-portfolios makes it possible to easily collect such events, return to them and analyse them in the light of new experiences. It may be more difficult to quickly locate such incidents in a paper journal unless you use some form of indexing system. Such important analysis of critical incidents will enhance your development and the likelihood of producing a successful portfolio.

Success in developing an e-portfolio can be quite a challenge if you are not technically minded or prefer to handwrite your reflective journal. However, as technology develops and electronic portfolios become more user-friendly, some of these barriers may disappear. For example, instead of typing up your journal you will be able to record and download your experiences to your portfolio from your mobile phone.

To be successful in this type of portfolio it is essential that you:

- attend training sessions so that you are fully aware of how to access and use all the functions associated with your portfolio;
- regularly allocate time to your portfolio development;
- record and reflect on critical incidents;
- ensure that you respond to feedback from your tutor so that you can demonstrate your ability to respond positively to criticism.

What are portfolios used to assess?

As we have seen in the preceding discussions, portfolios are used to assess a range of evidence based on your experience and learning. These may include:

- progression from one stage of your programme to another, for example, progressing from Year 1 to Year 2 of your programme;
- the completion of specific competencies;
- the development of specific skills;
- your ability to meet specific learning outcomes;
- your ability to recognise and learn from critical incidents;
- suitability for registration;
- suitability for a specific role/post;
- a combination of all or any of the above.

Portfolios require time and preparation if they are to be developed to a successful standard. Following are some points you will need to consider.

How can I be successful in portfolio assessments?

As with all assessments, time spent in preparation is the first step in producing a successful portfolio.

1. Access the learning outcomes that apply to your portfolio and ensure that you are clear about the content you will need to include.
2. Read the assessment guidelines and ensure you understand the format in which the portfolio is to be presented e.g. manual or electronic, number of sections.
3. Collect your evidence and set aside time to reflect on your achievements, disappointments and critical incidents so that you can include a well-thought-out action plan for your future personal and professional development.

Activity 5.2   *Evidence-based practice and research*

-   Access your programme handbook and identify assessments that require a portfolio to be completed.
-   Using the information you find, select the portfolio assessment you have to complete next.
-   Complete the activities in the three points given above this activity box so that you have completed the preparation for your portfolio.

As this activity is personal to you, there is no worked example at the end of the chapter.

With good preparation you will now be ready to compile and complete a successful portfolio. You should remember to:

-   include your name and/or candidate number;
-   ensure each section of your portfolio is clearly marked with a divider and labelled;
-   ensure the evidence you use is of good quality;
-   make clear links between the evidence you present and the learning outcomes;
-   ensure any reflection elements in your portfolio conclude with an action point for future personal and/or professional development.

Portfolio as a record of achievement

This type of portfolio has similarities to the *record of achievement* you may have been required to keep at school. It should contain evidence of your education and work achievements, and can be used to form the basis of a professional portfolio or profile.

> ## Case study: Ben
>
> *When Ben answered his phone this morning he was not expecting to be told he had gained his first post as a staff nurse. Ben had completed his nursing programme in a provincial hospital, but had always wanted to work in a London teaching hospital once qualified. When he attended the interview in London it had been obvious that competition for the post was significant. He was confident that he had done well in his maths test but wasn't sure if he had done enough in his interview to get the job. As he listened to the feedback from his new employer he realised that the time he had spent preparing his portfolio had been worthwhile and that the interview panel were impressed by the range and quality of evidence he was able to produce to demonstrate his student nursing experiences, which had included feedback from his mentors and service users.*

For Ben, maintaining a portfolio had begun at school with his *record of achievement*. At university he had been required to present a portfolio of evidence of his progression in theory and practice at the end of each academic year. He had found it easy to draw from these two types of portfolio to create a new one that reflected both his personal and professional development in preparation for his job interview. In this instance Ben has used his portfolio as a record of his achievements before and during his nursing programme.

Ben constructed his portfolio so that he could demonstrate his suitability for the post. He put himself in the shoes of the employer and sought the evidence needed to demonstrate his suitability for the post.

Concept summary: Post-registration education and practice (PREP)

The successful portfolio of evidence Ben has developed for his job interviews will form the foundation of the portfolio that all registered nurses are required to maintain in order to demonstrate their fitness to re-register as a nurse every three years. The NMC calls this type of portfolio a personal professional profile.

The prep handbook (NMC, 2011b) states:

> 12. *You must document, in your profile, your relevant learning activity and the way in which it has informed and influenced your practice . . .*

As you can see from this statement, producing a successful portfolio is not only important for progression on your nursing programme but also an essential feature of the maintenance of your professional registration and nursing career.

What is this type of portfolio used to assess?

Successful portfolios of this type are used to demonstrate that you have had sufficient experience, knowledge and skills to meet the demands of a specific role/post or the requirements for re-registration.

In terms of content it is important to include the following.

- An up-to-date CV that leads with your most recent academic award and nursing experience. Ensure that experience, knowledge and skills that are relevant to the role/post are prominent and not hidden after old and less relevant content.
- A summary of your practice placements so that it is easy for a prospective employer to gain an overall impression of practice experiences. Add a few lines of comment to each placement summary identifying specific learning you have gained from the placement.
- At the beginning a description of the placements most relevant to the role/post you are applying for.
- Copies of feedback from mentors and service users that will enable the prospective employer to see evidence of how others have seen the quality of care you deliver.
- A section describing any paid/voluntary work or additional training/courses you have been involved with since starting your nursing programme. This will indicate your willingness to take advantage of additional learning opportunities.
- A back section that can be used as a type of appendix where you can include original documents such as your completed practice documentation and academic feedback sheets.

Use your portfolio during the interview to evidence your suitability for the post. Having spent time developing this type of achievement portfolio, you will have reminded yourself of all the elements that have contributed to your development as a nurse, and this process will help you to respond to questions related to your suitability for the role/post you have applied for. This will contribute to the likelihood of a successful outcome.

Activity 5.3   *Decision-making*

Access a CV format. This may be one recommended by the careers department of your university. Use your chosen format to build your own professional CV that you can use when you begin to look for your first staff nurse post. Although most applications are now electronic and do not require you to send a CV, you can copy and paste information from your CV directly into your applications.

Time spent completing a CV and writing a brief statement of your knowledge, skills and qualities will enable you to be well prepared when job opportunities arise.

The Royal College of Nursing offers its student members advice on CV and portfolio production that you may find useful. The web address is included at the end of the chapter.

As this activity is focused on your own achievements, there is no example at the end of the chapter.

You will need to use your own judgement to produce a successful professional portfolio/profile as you will need to decide what specific achievements and interests you will make your main focus. Other types of portfolios will be more prescriptive and will require you to produce specific evidence to meet specific outcomes.

Activity 5.4   *Communication*

Let us return to Ben and the portfolio he had developed to support his job application.

What would you have included in your portfolio to take with you to interview? Provide a rationale for your decisions.

When you have completed this activity, compare your ideas with those listed at the end of the chapter.

Chapter summary

This chapter has considered the purpose of portfolios and what they might be used to assess. It has explored the principles you need to address if you are to produce a successful portfolio. It has stressed the importance of reflecting on critical incidents in order to demonstrate your ability to think critically about your experiences and learn from them.

Activities: brief outline answers

Activity 5.1: Critical thinking (page 67)

Identifying the cause of Amy's lack of confidence will be central to developing an effective plan.

In the SWOT analysis given in Table 5.1, Amy identifies assertive communication as the main area for development. In the worked example below it is assumed that Amy's lack of confidence has its basis in her difficulty understanding some aspects of altered physiology and drug calculations so that a different action plan can be considered.

For this alternative action plan Amy could identify the following goals.

- Identify the type of conditions I will meet on next placements. Make a list of these conditions and a revision timetable. Revise the related altered physiology in preparation for and during my placement.
- Discuss with my mentor the altered physiology of patients in my care and link to their nursing care and medication management.
- Practise drug calculations using the university online programme and drug calculation book. Practise drug calculations for my patients each shift. Once I can consistently correctly calculate straightforward drug calculations, progress to calculating more complex prescriptions.

Activity 5.4: Communication (page 75)

CV content	Rationale
Personal and contact information	Make sure that you include your postcode and contact details. Create a professional email address that is separate from your personal account. Some personal email addresses are not suitable for professional correspondence, e.g. a hotmail address such as suzyboo@hotmail.co.uk may create the wrong impression.
Details of nursing programme and predicted degree classification.	By identifying some details of your nursing education you can present the aspects of your nursing programme you consider to be particularly good. Your academic achievement will be of particular interest if the post you are applying for may lead to future study at Masters level, e.g. public health nursing.
Other academic qualifications.	Be brief here. For example, 4 A levels grade AABC (Biology, Psychology, French and Maths); 10 CGSE grades A-C (English, Maths, French, Biology, Psychology, Sociology, Art, etc.).
Summary of placement experience during programme and the learning outcomes achieved as a result.	Completing a summary table of your practice experience will enable your prospective employer to gain an overview of your experience at a glance. Be sure to place first the most relevant to the post and the most recent experience, and note the knowledge and skills gained for each placement. Do not use the name of units, hospital or Trusts but instead give a general description, e.g. medical assessment unit, district nursing.
Statement of personal attributes, professional skills and interests.	Produce a picture of the type of person you are. This could include terms such as conscientious, hard working and team player. Be prepared to give examples to support these statements and why you have developed specific areas of interest.
Paid/voluntary work undertaken while at university.	Only include this here if it is health-related work.
Summary of previous work experience under generic headings, e.g. retails, management, administration.	Only include work experience that is relevant. If you have had a variety of jobs in retail or catering, then group them under these headings and identify what skills you have developed that can be useful in your nursing career, e.g. customer service.

Other elements of your portfolio would include the following.

Copies of mentor and service user comments.	This provides evidence of your development as a professional and the quality of the care you provide.
Critical incident analysis.	Inclusion of this form of reflective learning demonstrates your ability to learn from practice experience.
Feedback sheets from assignments.	Provides additional information on your academic abilities.
Appendix of evidence.	You should include original documents in this section, such as original practice documentation, education certificates and results from annual examination boards.

Further reading

Howatson-Jones, L (2010) *Reflective practice in nursing.* Exeter: Learning Matters.

This excellent book provides a clear introduction to the process of reflection and the use of models of reflection.

Hutchfield, K (2010) *Information skills for nursing.* Exeter: Learning Matters.

This book provides an introduction to professional development planning and the SBAR model of communication.

Reed, S (2011) *Success with your professional portfolio for nursing students.* Exeter: Learning Matters.

This book offers an introduction to developing a range of portfolios used in nursing.

Useful website

www.rcn.org.uk/development/learning/learningzone

If you are a member of the Royal College of Nursing, this site offers access to some very useful guidance on CV writing and portfolio development.

Chapter 6
Succeeding in Objective Structured Clinical Examinations (OSCEs)

Pam Page

NMC Standards for Pre-registration Nursing Education

This chapter will address the following competencies:

Domain 1: Professional values

1. All nurses must practise with confidence according to *The code: Standards of conduct, performance and ethics for nurses and midwives* (NMC, 2008), and within other recognised ethical and legal frameworks. They must be able to recognise and address ethical challenges relating to people's choices and decision-making about their care, and act within the law to help them and their families and carers find acceptable solutions.

Domain 2: Communication and interpersonal skills

4. All nurses must recognise when people are anxious or in distress and respond effectively, using therapeutic principles, to promote their wellbeing, manage personal safety and resolve conflict. They must use effective communication strategies and negotiation techniques to achieve best outcomes, respecting the dignity and human rights of all concerned. They must know when to consult a third party and how to make referrals for advocacy, mediation or arbitration.

Domain 3: Nursing practice and decision-making

2. All nurses must possess a broad knowledge of the structure and functions of the human body, and other relevant knowledge from the life, behavioural and social sciences as applied to health, ill health, disability, ageing and death. They must have an in-depth knowledge of common physical and mental health problems and treatments in their own field of practice, including co-morbidity and physiological and psychological vulnerability.

NMC Essential Skills Clusters

This chapter will address the following ESCs:

Cluster: Care, compassion and communication

1. As partners in the care process, people can trust a newly registered graduate nurse to provide collaborative care based on the highest standards, knowledge and competence.

continued . . .

3. People can trust the newly registered graduate nurse to respect them as individuals and strive to help them preserve their dignity at all times.

Cluster: Organisational aspects of care

9. People can trust the newly registered graduate nurse to treat them as partners and work with them to make a holistic and systematic assessment of their needs; to develop a personalised plan that is based on mutual understanding and respect for their individual situation promoting health and well-being, minimising risk of harm and promoting their safety at all times.

10. People can trust the newly registered graduate nurse to deliver nursing interventions and evaluate their effectiveness against the agreed assessment and care plan.

18. People can trust a newly registered graduate nurse to enhance the safety of service users and identify and actively manage risk and uncertainty in relation to people, the environment, self and others.

Cluster: Infection prevention and control

21. People can trust the newly registered graduate nurse to identify and take effective measures to prevent and control infection in accordance with local and national policy.

Chapter aims

By the end of this chapter you should be able to:

*   understand what the acronym OSCE stands for and the key features of an OSCE;
*   know what to expect from an OSCE and how to prepare for the OSCE performance;
*   gain insight into the OSCE experience from both a student and examiner perspective;
*   be able to formulate a plan to assist you with OSCE preparation and success;
*   reflect and learn from the OSCE experience.

Introduction

Anne, a first-year undergraduate student nurse, discovers that she has a summative assessment involving an OSCE in her module handbook. Anne has never heard of the acronym OSCE. What should she do?

She should read this chapter, which will not only explain the term OSCE but will also explain why OSCEs are increasingly being used as both formative and summative assessment in pre-registration nursing degree programmes and, more importantly, help you to prepare for and successfully complete an OSCE.

If you are in the same situation as Anne, you may feel anxious about the prospect of being examined in a simulation situation. This chapter will guide you through what an OSCE is and why they are used. It will prepare you for the assessment and help identify top tips for success. Finally, it will support you in learning from the whole OSCE experience.

The OSCE acronym

The term OSCE is an acronym that stands for Objective Structured Clinical Examination. Watson et al. (2002, p424) describes the OSCE as an exam where *students demonstrate their competence under a variety of simulated conditions.* What does this mean for Anne? Essentially, she will be required to perform specific skills (with underpinning knowledge) together with appropriate behaviour within a clinical skills laboratory that reflects a patient care environment. This is sometimes known as 'knowing, showing and doing' – the building blocks of competence.

OSCEs have been used for many years in medical and dental education (Rushforth, 2007) but are increasingly being used in nursing, midwifery and other allied health professions. OSCEs may also be referred to as OSCLAs (Objective Structured Clinical Learning Assessments) but the essential components are the same.

Why are OSCEs being used as a form of assessment?

Your university is required to demonstrate that you are fit for purpose and practice at the end of your three-year programme (NMC, 2008). Historically, an apprenticeship model of training was used, and frequently the evidence base for practice was missing, putting patient safety at risk. The introduction of simulated learning within universities (skills laboratories) allows you to develop clinical skills in a safe environment; these skills can then be transferred to the clinical setting with much greater confidence and competence. The format of OSCEs can vary between universities; you may have a number of short 'stations' (dedicated areas in the skills laboratory), each assessing a different clinical skill, or one station where a number of skills are assessed. The type of clinical skill assessed in Year 1 may relate to patient communication, patient assessment and infection control. Year 2 may contain skills stations relating to medicine administration, and Year 3 will contain more complex patient scenarios. Examples of these will be identified throughout the chapter. Be assured that the type of skills station will be appropriate to your stage of education.

OSCEs can be used both formatively and summatively (refer to Chapter 1 to understand the nature of formative and summative assessment), and while they can create a high level of anxiety they also generate a higher level of confidence in the clinical setting (Nulty et al., 2011).

What areas of practice may be assessed by OSCE?

OSCEs are a form of assessment that allow you to demonstrate your clinical skills (psychomotor domain), knowledge (cognitive domain) and attitude (affective domain). This style of simulation allows skill assessment and demonstration of your knowledge and attitude in a safe and professional environment. You may be assessed formatively to help you identify strengths and weaknesses in your performance or summatively as part of passing progression points within the programme.

Skills commonly assessed in the first year of your undergraduate nursing programme include:

- hand hygiene;
- communication skills;
- basic life support;
- clinical observations (pulse, blood pressure, respiratory rate, temperature);
- medicine administration.

In your second and third years, scenarios will become more complex and integrated, e.g. assessing a deteriorating patient.

Activity 6.1   *Evidence-based practice and research*

Take a few minutes to consider how you measure a radial pulse. Jot down some notes.

An outline answer is given at the end of the chapter.

Did you consider the following points?

- Having the necessary equipment (fob watch with second hand and observation chart).
- Importance of universal precautions and hand hygiene.
- Explaining the procedure and obtaining consent from the patient.
- Where to locate the radial pulse using the first and second fingers.
- How to count the pulse rate for one minute, including assessment of rhythm and regularity as well as rate.
- Accurate documentation and escalating concern (if appropriate).

It should become apparent to you that there are many facets to performing this skill. Not only are you demonstrating knowledge regarding anatomy and physiology, but also understanding why you are recording the pulse as well as performing the skill itself. When performed in context, it will also demonstrate communication with the patient, documenting the pulse rate and interpreting the result. In essence, you will need to demonstrate not only skill performance, but also the correct knowledge and behaviour in the context of the clinical situation.

Think!

- Knowledge (cognitive domain).
- Skill (psychomotor domain).
- Attitude (affective domain).
- Context.

Knowledge	Anatomy and physiology of radial artery, normal pulse rate and the implications of deviation from the normal range.
Skill	Demonstrates universal precautions; locates and records pulse rate, volume and regularity accurately.
	Establishes rapport, explains procedure, gains consent, i.e. communicates effectively.
Attitude	Shows respect for patient dignity, and demonstrates care and compassion throughout.
Context	This is important as it will determine escalation and communication of any concerns, e.g. are you in the hospital car park, on community placement or in the Emergency Department?

So now that Anne knows what an OSCE is and why they are being used on her programme, we need to support her through the process of successfully completing her OSCE.

How to prepare for OSCEs

Within the nursing profession there are some essential principles that underpin our performance and behaviour in clinical practice.

Activity 6.2   *Evidence-based practice and research*

Spend a few minutes identifying what professional guidelines and policies underpin clinical practice in relation to recording a radial pulse.

An outline answer is given at the end of the chapter.

In essence, there are five core principles that underpin safe clinical practice (Bloomfield et al., 2010).

- Infection control.
- Evidence-based practice.

- Accurate documentation and record keeping.
- Effective communication.
- Maintaining dignity and respect.

Apply these to your OSCE and you are well on the way to success.

Preparation is the key to success

There is no question that undertaking an OSCE will generate a level of anxiety. Remember that some stress will enhance your performance, but excessive anxiety will inhibit your performance (Bloomfield et al., 2010). Nulty et al. (2011) evaluated the OSCE experience of 58 undergraduate student nurses: 88 per cent stated that they were *very nervous*; however, 79 per cent stated that *the examiner made me feel at ease*. Remember that assessors *want you to succeed*, but you must demonstrate competence in performing the skill in all domains (cognitive, affective and psychomotor).

Activity 6.3   *Reflection*

Reflect on previous examinations and formal assessments. Describe how you felt prior to these events and what strategies you used to minimise nerves and enhance your performance.

As this activity is based on your own reflection, there is no outline answer at the end of the chapter.

While there are no right or wrong answers to this activity, it is important that *you* know how you respond to stress to optimise your performance. If you experience panic sensations prior to assessments, then consider how you are going to address this. Simple breathing strategies can be helpful or spending the waiting time on your own to prepare yourself mentally for the assessment. Actually visualising yourself undertaking the OSCE and thinking about what you may be required to do and how you will respond has been shown to be useful (Bloomfield et al., 2010). Some universities have available to students vodcasts or video recordings of OSCEs that have been performed to a high standard. These are recordings of OSCEs undertaken by other students demonstrating 'best practice'. This allows students to become familiar with the format of OSCEs and may help in the visualisation process.

OSCE countdown

Guidance regarding the nature of the OSCE station you are required to undertake should be contained within your module handbook. This should also include the marking criteria – make sure that you familiarise yourself with both the guidance and the marking criteria. Knowing *what is expected of you and how you will be marked* is essential. OSCEs are frequently video recorded for moderation (to ensure marking is fair and accurate) and quality assurances purposes. Your consent should be obtained for this, and while it may provoke further anxiety, it does ensure that there is an accurate record of your performance and that any marking discrepancies are eliminated. You should also establish:

- what skills and knowledge are being assessed;
- how many skills stations there are;
- the duration of each skill station;
- how you will gain feedback on your performance.

At this stage you should be familiar with the underpinning theory for your OSCE assessment as well as policies and national drivers, and you should be able to cite these if requested by the examiner or produce a word-processed reference list according to your university's guidelines for submission at the OSCE.

Practise, practise, practise your skill in the skills laboratory under supervision, and discuss with your mentor in clinical practice. Many universities offer the opportunity to undertake mock OSCEs with feedback – this is an excellent opportunity to gain formative feedback on your performance and 'feel' the level of anxiety you may experience. Alternatively, book some time in the skills laboratories with your peer group and test each other on performing skills; ask each other what the evidence base is and provide constructive criticism on each other's overall performance.

Demonstrating a professional attitude throughout the OSCE is essential. From the initial meeting with the patient and gaining consent through to explanation of procedures and final closure of the OSCE, a professional behaviour needs to be evidenced. In other words, you must demonstrate professional behaviour from beginning to end.

There are some practical aspects of preparation too.

- Allow time to prepare mentally and physically on the day of the OSCE.
- Ensure you get a good night's sleep.
- Check where the OSCEs are to be held, what time you must arrive and whether you need to wear your uniform.

In addition, there may be practical items that you need to bring with you, for example:

- student ID card with SID number and photo;
- watch with second hand.

If uniform is required, ensure your uniform complies with uniform policy.

Activity 6.4   *Decision-making*

Write a preparation plan for your OSCE, including dates, times and location. As well as considering practical aspects, schedule in time for psychological preparation.

An outline answer is given at the end of the chapter.

Top ten tips for success

1. Get organised.
2. Understand the assessment.
3. Start preparing well in advance of the summative assessment.
4. Review lecture notes and relevant texts/policies.
5. Get answers to your questions.
6. Quiz yourself and rehearse answers out loud.
7. Find a friend or form a study group – practise mock OSCEs and give honest but constructive feedback.
8. Attend formative OSCEs and preparatory sessions.
9. Relax – eat and sleep well in the knowledge that you *are* prepared for your OSCE.
10. Reflect and learn from the experience.

The OSCE experience

The OSCE process is very formal, which may surprise you, but remember that it is an examination and examination conditions, e.g. timing, will be strictly applied. If you undertake more than one skills station, you may find one harder than others – just like exam questions – but you must move on from one station to the next in the allotted timeframe.

You should be aware that a variety of simulated clients can be used at OSCE stations. They may include:

- manikins (basic and high fidelity);
- clinical staff;
- actors;
- members of the public;
- academic staff and/or students.

Whichever model is used, you must remember to apply professional principles of dignity, respect, care, compassion and communication throughout your time at each of the skills stations (NMC, 2010c).

All student nurses (irrespective of their field of nursing) are required to be competent in basic life support (BLS) prior to their first practice placement. You, like Anne, may be required to undertake an OSCE in BLS. She will be provided with guidelines (see below) in advance of the actual assessment together with marking criteria. OSCEs can be marked on a pass/fail basis, graded (A, B, C, etc.) or fine graded by percentage.

OSCE guidelines (example)

The purpose of this OSCE is to assess the knowledge and skill required to effectively care for a patient in cardiac arrest according to the UK Resuscitation Council 2010 guidelines. The OSCE will consist of two skills stations. The first will require you to recognise and treat a manikin in cardiac arrest (five minutes). The second will be a short multiple choice paper (MCQ) to assess your knowledge of BLS (ten minutes).

Marking criteria will include:

* recognition of safe environment;
* recognising the unconscious patient;
* calling for help;
* airway skills, including use of 'pocket mask';
* competent cardiac massage.

On arrival at the OSCE skills station Anne will be provided with a scenario (see below) to contextualise her assessment. She should read this carefully and seek clarification from the examiner if she is unclear about what is required.

Scenario

You are a first-year student nurse on placement in the community. Your mentor is attending to the patient, who has a leg ulcer. You hear a loud thud from the next room and go to investigate. The patient's partner has collapsed on the floor, is unresponsive and going blue. Please assess the situation, articulate your findings and demonstrate what action you would take.

While you are undertaking your OSCE, the examiner will be assessing your performance using a checklist of criteria. It is not uncommon for another examiner, known as a *moderator*, also to be in the room. Do not allow yourself to be distracted by the presence of moderators or external examiners – remember that this is to ensure that the assessment process is fair and objective.

OSCE examiners often comment that it is always easy to distinguish between students who have prepared for their OSCE and those who have not. So make sure you have undertaken the preparation, and remember that if things do start to go wrong, tell the examiner. That way, they will be able to make a judgement about whether your practice is safe. Say nothing and you could fail through unsafe practice.

Activity 6.5   *Decision-making*

Now is a good time to reflect on what you have learnt about OSCEs and to note down how you feel about your impending OSCE.

As this activity is based on your own reflection, there is no outline answer at the end of the chapter

You may still feel anxious about OSCEs; however, you should be aware that students have clearly benefited from the 'OSCE experience'.

There is good evidence that once you have successfully completed your OSCE you will feel more confident about your clinical practice. Students have made the following comments about their OSCE experience:

> *This OSCE has increased my confidence for what may be coming next year.*
> (Nulty et al., 2011)

> *I feel more confident because I can actually demonstrate the basic assessment skills.*
> (Nulty et al., 2011)

> *Doing an OSCE really did make a difference to my learning and practice. Passing the OSCE gave me a huge sense of pride in my practice.*
> (Bloomfield et al., 2010)

This demonstrates that OSCEs are not just about assessment but do actually aid learning.

Life after your first OSCE

OSCEs are as much about *your learning* as passing an assessment within your programme. As such, you need to:

- recognise good performance;
- develop your reflective skills;
- understand and use feedback effectively.

If you failed your OSCE, you need to be fully aware of the consequences. If the exam was formative, then the result is important but not as final as with a summative assessment. An important outcome is that you can recognise your performance level and how it needs to be improved. If you have failed a summative OSCE, you *must* seek tutorial support prior to your second attempt. You will receive written feedback on your performance. Lecturers will normally offer remedial workshops in skill laboratories for you to rehearse. It is vital that you reflect on your own performance and recognise your strengths and weaknesses. There are several reflective tools that can support you in this – you may wish to refer to *Reflective practice in nursing* (Howatson-Jones, 2010), which is part of the *Transforming Nursing Practice* series. Plan your revision strategy – try writing an action plan to maximise your chances of success.

Whatever the outcome of your OSCE, it is important that you utilise the learning. You may have been surprised at your own actions and reactions during the actual OSCE.

Activity 6.6   *Decision-making*

As the final activity of this chapter, write some notes on your own performance, clearly identifying what you have learnt and what learning deficits remain. How will you use your OSCE experience to aid future learning?

An outline answer is given at the end of the chapter.

OSCEs can never be seen in isolation, as they are the building blocks for your whole nursing programme. You will be applying these skills in clinical practice and developing them into an ever expanding portfolio of professional knowledge, skills and behaviours.

Chapter summary

This chapter has introduced you to assessment by OSCE, an increasingly used mode of assessment within nursing degrees that crosses all fields. We have established what an OSCE is, why it is used and how OSCEs can increase in complexity through your degree programme. We have talked through how to prepare effectively for success in your OSCE and what to expect when you walk into your OSCE station. Finally, we have identified the benefits of assessment by OSCE, notably an increase in confidence in clinical practice, and emphasised the importance of reflecting and learning from the experience.

Activities: brief outline answers

Activity 6.1: Evidence-based practice and research (page 81)

You may have included the following points.

- Equipment required: fob watch, observation chart.
- Universal precautions and hand hygiene.
- Accurate documentation and escalation.

Full details on undertaking this skill can be obtained from *The Royal Marsden Hospital manual of clinical nursing procedures*, 8th edition, p749 (Dougherty and Lister, 2011). Refer also to your local Trust policy on clinical observations.

Activity 6.2: Evidence-based practice and research (page 82)

You may have included the following points.

- *The code: Standards of conduct, performance and ethics for nurses and midwives* (NMC, 2008).
- *NICE Clinical Guideline 50: Acutely ill patients in hospital* (NICE, 2007).
- *Infection control: prevention of healthcare-associated infection in primary and community care* (NICE, 2003).

- Mental Capacity Act (Department of Health, 2005).
- *Essence of care* benchmarks (Department of Health, 2007).

Activity 6.4: Decision-making (page 84)

You may have included the following points.

- Date, time, place and venue of OSCE.
- Travel arrangements.
- Skills and knowledge to be assessed.
- Resources to use – websites, lecture notes, journal articles, textbooks.
- Countdown plan – one month before, one week before, the day before and the day of the OSCE.
- Study group – share contact details and arrange to meet.

Activity 6.6: Decision-making (page 87)

You may have included the following points.

- Using a reflective model to identify learning points.
- Identifying the strengths of your performance from the feedback, building on these and celebrating them.
- Identifying the weaknesses of your performance and filling the gaps, remembering to identify whether the gap is knowledge (cognitive), skills (psychomotor), attitude (affective) or related to the clinical context.
- Identifying what you have learnt about yourself and how this will influence future performance.

Further reading

Cabellaro, C and Creed, F (2012) *Nursing OSCEs: a complete guide to exam success.* Oxford: Oxford University Press.

This book provides further detailed information on preparing for the ten most common OSCE stations undertaken by nursing students.

Merriman, C and Westcott, E (2010) *Succeed in OSCEs and practical exams: an essential guide for nurses.* London: McGraw Hill.

This book specifies how to prepare successfully for all practice-based nursing assessments.

Chapter 7
Succeeding in presentations

Kay Hutchfield

NMC Standards for Pre-registration Nursing Education

This chapter will address the following competencies:

Domain 1: Professional values

6. All nurses must understand the roles and responsibilities of other health and social care professionals, and seek to work with them collaboratively for the benefit of all who need care.

Domain 2: Communication and interpersonal skills

2. All nurses must use a range of communication skills and technologies to support person-centred care and enhance quality and safety. They must ensure people receive all the information they need in a language and manner that allows them to make informed choices and share decision-making. They must recognise when language interpretation or other communication support is needed and know how to obtain it.

Domain 3: Nursing practice and decision-making

2. All nurses must possess a broad knowledge of the structure and functions of the human body, and other relevant knowledge from the life, behavioural and social sciences as applied to health, ill health, disability, ageing and death. They must have an in-depth knowledge of common physical and mental health problems and treatments in their own field of practice, including co-morbidity and physiological and psychological vulnerability.

Domain 4: Leadership, management and team working

6. All nurses must work independently as well as in teams. They must be able to take the lead in coordinating, delegating and supervising care safely, managing risk and remaining accountable for the care given.

NMC Essential Skills Clusters

This chapter will address the following ESCs:

Cluster: Care, compassion and communication

4. People can trust a newly qualified graduate nurse to engage with them and their family or carers within their cultural environments in an acceptant and anti-discriminatory manner free from harassment and exploitation.

continued . . .

By the first progression point:

ii.   Respects people's rights.

By entry to the register:

vii. Manages and diffuses challenging situations effectively.

Cluster: Organisational aspects of care

12. People can trust the newly registered graduate nurse to respond to their feedback and a wide range of other sources to learn, develop and improve services.

By the second progression point:

iii. Uses supervision and other forms of reflective learning to make effective use of feedback.

By entry to the register:

vi.   Actively responds to feedback.

15. People can trust the newly registered graduate nurse to safely delegate to others and to respond appropriately when a task is delegated to them.

By the first progression point:

i.   Accepts delegated activities within limitations of own role, knowledge and skill.

Chapter aims

By the end of this chapter you should be able to:

* identify the core principles of successful individual and group presentations;
* understand how presentations can contribute to the development of practice competencies.

Introduction

Case study: Group presentation

Sam is a first-year nursing student and contributed to a group seminar as part of an inter-professional practice module. She was allocated to a group that consisted of four other nursing students: a radiography student, two occupational therapy students and a midwifery student. The group had decided on the content of their presentation and divided up the topic into four discrete sections. Sam had never done a presentation before and was a little anxious as she was also allocated to work with another adult nursing student, Jade, who she had not met before. They made arrangements to meet in the library to work together on their section of the group presentation. On the day of each arranged meeting Jade either texted Sam with an excuse as to why she could

continued . . .

not make the meeting or arrived late when Sam had completed most of the work. Sam found it difficult to challenge Jade's behaviour, which resulted in her doing most of the work on her own and attending the presentation rehearsal without Jade.

On the day of the assessed presentation Jade announced that she would introduce their section of the presentation. Sam agreed to this but then Jade proceeded to present their whole section, even though it was apparent that her understanding of the topic was poor. Sam was left with little to add. She felt stupid in front of her peers and tutor as it seemed as if she had contributed little to the work of the group. This assumption was also reflected in the peer and tutor evaluation and feedback.

Sam's group was allocated a borderline pass mark, the lowest mark of all the groups presenting.

Activity 7.1   *Communication and team working*

From this experience, what lessons do you think Sam learnt about participating in a successful group presentation? How could she avoid a repetition of this situation in future group presentations?

Compare your thoughts with those at the end of the chapter.

Individual and group oral, visual and audio-visual presentations will feature as both formative and summative assessments within your nursing programme. They offer an alternative means of assessment to written assignments and examinations, and provide the opportunity for students to demonstrate their ability to effectively communicate information orally and visually as well as in writing. To be successful in presentations you will need to consider three main elements: preparation, delivery and feedback. Before we move on to these elements, it is important to consider what skills you might need to develop in order to undertake a successful presentation.

Activity 7.2   *Reflection and critical thinking*

Take a moment to consider the skills you need to undertake successful presentations.

Make a list of these skills; highlighting any you feel you need to develop further.

How might the skills you have developed through giving presentations be useful in your clinical practice as a student and qualified nurse?

Compare your thoughts with those at the end of the chapter.

Effective preparation for your presentation

To be effective in your preparation for your presentation you need to consider a number of factors.

1. The learning outcomes or the learning task that needs to be achieved.
2. The location/environment in which the presentation will be given.
3. The required presentation style.
4. The allocated time.
5. The audience.
6. Handouts and other resources.

1. The learning outcomes or the learning task that needs to be achieved

This is the most important element of preparation for any assignment. If you do not focus your presentation on what is required, you place yourself at risk of failing your presentation. In Chapter 2, we discussed how summative assessments are designed to measure whether or not you have met the learning outcomes for an element of intended learning for a module or course. Some summative and formative assessments may take the form of a presentation, so to ensure success it is essential that you are clear about the purpose of the presentation and the topic area that needs to be included. If in doubt, read the assignment guidelines and marking criteria, and then check your understanding with the tutor responsible for assessing your presentation.

As with written assignments, it is important to gain a good understanding of the topic and then to select out the key elements that you wish to include in your presentation. You may find it useful to return to Chapter 2 and revisit the content from the end of Activity 2.3 to the end of Activity 2.6 so that you have an effective timeline for preparing a successful presentation.

2. The location

The location for your presentation will determine the most effective presentation style to use.

Case study: Practice teaching

Jess is a third-year children's nursing student and as part of her current placement she is required to develop a presentation for three first-year students that will be formatively assessed by her mentor. She will use feedback from this formative assessment to write a reflection on the development of her teaching skills.

She has agreed with her mentor that her presentation will focus attention on teaching the students about the normal ranges of pulse and respirations in children and how to take a pulse and respiratory rate. Jess is quite confident about using PowerPoint and has used it to develop her presentation and handout. However, when making enquiries about using the unit laptop and projector she discovers they are already booked out to someone else.

Activity 7.3 *Critical thinking and decision-making*

Reflect on how Jess could modify/adapt her presentation so that she can deliver it success-fully in practice environment.

What else could Jess do to maximise the effectiveness of her presentation?

An outline answer is given at the end of the chapter.

As you can see from the scenario, technology is not always available. You must therefore be familiar with the location in which your presentation will take place so that you can develop your presentation accordingly. Technical failure is always a possibility and you should be prepared for this. For example, as well as having a copy of your presentation on your pen drive, you could send a copy to your university email so that you can access it easily if your pen drive fails or is lost. It is also important to maximise the use of any resources available in the location that could be used to enhance your presentation.

Noise and possible interruptions are factors to take into account when planning your presen-tation. Summative presentations will take place in a university setting, and your tutor will be responsible for ensuring that you have a suitable room, as examination conditions will apply during summative presentation assessments. It is important to make time to check the layout of the room in which your presentation will take place so that you can decide where to stand so that the audience can see you as well as the screen, can make sure you are familiar with the equipment.

In the practice setting it may be more challenging to reduce noise and avoid interruptions that can impact on the effectiveness of your presentation. In these situations you need to be aware that noise and interruptions may interfere with the transfer of information and ensure that you check that the information you are providing has been understood.

3. The required presentation style

The style of presentation will be dependent on whether it is an individual or group presentation and will be clearly identified in the assignment guidelines. This section will consider three common formats for presentations: PowerPoint, posters and group presentation (including role play).

Before moving on to explore the specific requirements of these three formats it is important to consider what you have already learnt from your own experiences of giving or attending a presentation.

Activity 7.4 *Critical thinking and decision-making*

Reflect on good and poor presentations you have given and/or witnessed. Think about the factors that have influenced the way you felt about the presentation and make a list of dos and don'ts that you consider important for a successful presentation.

---

continued . . .

As we work through the various types of presentations, add to your list of dos and don'ts.

Armed with your expanded list of dos and don'ts, you will have identified those factors that will influence your presentation style and contribute to making your presentation successful.

This activity is continued in Activity 7.5, so there is no outline answer at the end of the chapter at this stage.

Delivering a successful presentation

PowerPoint presentations

It is quite possible that you have experienced both stimulating and boring PowerPoint presentations. The term 'death by PowerPoint' is often associated with a boring presentation delivered in a monotone and where the presenter merely reads the content of each slide to the audience. It is important that you avoid this style of PowerPoint presentation if you wish to complete a successful presentation.

PowerPoint may be used to successfully present a case study, for example. Within this type of presentation you may be required to demonstrate your knowledge and understanding of specific aspects of a patient/client journey. This may include, for example, altered physiology, pharmacology, nursing and communication.

To produce a successful presentation there are some principles you will need to apply.

*   *Gain and keep the attention of your audience.* This can be achieved by speaking clearly and confidently and making eye contact with the audience. The use of visual or audio cues at the start of your presentation can be very effective in gaining attention. Trying to keep your voice lively will also help. Know your audience so that you use language that is appropriate. For example, you should not use lay terms in a presentation to nursing students, e.g. tummy instead of abdomen.
*   *Clearly state the purpose of your presentation.* Making the purpose of your presentation clear at the beginning will not only help your audience to follow your presentation, but will also help you to keep focused on your topic.
*   *Include accurate and current knowledge/evidence.* You will not be successful in your presentation unless your knowledge is sound and up to date, and you are able to apply knowledge to your practice. It is not enough just to show what you know about a topic (descriptive knowledge – p6); you will also have to offer an ability to analyse and apply your knowledge. The author and year of publication should be included on each slide to demonstrate that you have used appropriate sources of information to inform your presentation. A full reference list of these sources should be provided at the end of the presentation in the form of a handout.
*   *Ensure the audience can read, see and hear the presentation.* If the audience cannot read your slides because the slides are too crowded with text or the font is too small, it will detract attention from your presentation. Remember to restrict the slide content to key points that you can talk to rather than just put all you want to say on to the slide. The colour you choose for the text

and background is also important. A white or pale-coloured font against a light background will be difficult to read from a distance. Avoid using capital letters other than at the beginning of sentences or for proper nouns, as a whole sentence or heading written in capital letters is difficult to read. Using cards with notes and cues can make you feel more confident, but remember to secure them together so if you drop them they will stay in order.

- *Animation.* PowerPoint presentations offer a range of graphics, templates and animations designed to enhance your presentation. However, it is possible to become too absorbed in this aspect of the presentation at a cost to the time needed to develop content or practise delivery. Only add features that will enhance understanding and interest or your presentation may become more about your ability to use resources available through PowerPoint than about the academic content. If you have inserted hyperlinks in your presentation, check they work and that there is internet access available if the link is to an online source.

- *Keep to agreed timeframe.* To be successful in a summative assessment you will need to keep within the allocated time. As in examinations you will be required to stop at a particular time and will not be allowed to continue, even if you have not finished your presentation. Failing to complete the presentation will obviously reduce the mark you are awarded. The key to keeping to time is to practise (ideally with a friend/relative as an audience). Talking faster is not the answer to having too much content as you will not allow your audience time to assimilate the information you are presenting. Presentations provide you with the opportunity for practising how to be concise when communicating important information to others. This is a very important skill to acquire for practice so that you are clear and concise in your communications with fellow professionals and service users.

Activity 7.5   *Reflection and critical thinking*

Presenting to your fellow students and tutor in a summative assessment can be daunting. Take a few minutes to finalise the list of dos and don'ts you began to construct in Activity 7.4. Consider what actions you have taken or could take that would allow you to feel and appear more confident when delivering a summative presentation.

Compare your ideas with those listed at the end of the chapter.

Knowing how to present yourself is a skill that is not just reserved for formal presentations; it will be very important to you when you are looking for your first staff nurse post. Although you may not be required to deliver a presentation at interview, you will need to present yourself as confident and a clear communicator, all skills that can be acquired through successful presentations in university.

We will now move on to the topic of poster presentation. This is a very useful skill to learn as, once qualified, you may wish to use this method to present practice development and research you have been engaged in. It will also be useful to you in your everyday work, for example, when producing service-user information or health-promotion posters.

Poster presentations

A poster is a visual representation of something that should relay a message without the need for the spoken word. The design should allow it to be read from a distance of three to five feet. It will be important for you to read the poster presentation guidelines to ensure that you produce a poster that is in the correct size and format for your assessment.

The key elements of a successful poster presentation are outlined below.

1. Text is large enough to be seen from five feet away and is kept to a minimum. A general guide is 40–48 font size for title and 24 minimum font size for other content. However, note that if you are producing your poster on A4 paper and then plan to enlarge it to A3 or A1, this will also increase the font size.
2. The visual appearance/layout draws the eye of the audience to it and generates interest.
3. Around 40 per cent of the poster is blank, giving an uncluttered appearance.
4. The purpose of the poster is clear and the content and sequence self-explanatory.
5. Only key information/themes are included.
6. Illustrations, images, graphs and diagrams are simple and clear (edited or cropped to remove unnecessary detail).
7. Background colours are neutral rather than bright.
8. Fonts and colours are used in a way that enhances understanding of the core message of the poster (no more than three colours if possible).
9. All illustrations, images, graphs and diagrams are clearly labelled and the sources are acknowledged and do not breach copyright.
10. Separate additional written information is provided along with a reference list of the material used to inform the development of the poster.

In assessed poster presentations you will be expected to have sufficient knowledge of the topic of your poster to respond to any questions from your fellow students or tutor.

Case study: Poster presentation

Hannah is a second-year mental health nursing student. She has just finished a placement in a Child and Adolescent Mental Health Service (CAMHS) unit. During her time in the unit she became aware of the impact domestic violence can have on children and how this can impact on their mental health and ability to achieve their full potential in adult life. She has decided to present this topic for her poster presentation.

Hannah has already read a considerable amount about domestic violence and has developed a comprehensive reference list and notes from which she plans to develop her poster. She decides on the title The impact of domestic violence on children *and uses a picture of a frightened child for the centre of her poster. Beneath the picture she has printed a short quote from a UNICEF report (2006),* For too many children, home is far from a safe haven. *Next to this she adds a simple graph that indicates the incidence of domestic violence in the UK. She decides to add a bullet-point list of the impact domestic violence has on children, and she positions it between the main heading and the central picture. She adds some texts on the long-term effects on*

continued . . .

adult health. In the last section she summarises the information from government guidelines on supporting children who are experiencing domestic violence. She uses headings and colour to make each section easy to identify and gives the title How can you help? *to the section on the government guidelines. By using the same colour box and the same size font, she hopes to focus her audience on positive action they can take to make a difference to children.*

From this case study you can see that the written content of the poster is not extensive and only key information is included. Once Hannah has completed this work on her poster, she can now focus on ensuring that she has achieved the focus she wants and can spend time adjusting colour, font and font size until she is happy with the visual effect of her poster.

One thing Hannah has thought about is whether any of her audience may themselves have experienced domestic violence as a child or be currently in an abusive relationship. She decides to make a small number of business-sized printed cards containing the contact details of local groups offering support to victims of domestic violence. She leaves the cards next to the poster with her handouts so that anyone who may need support can pick up a card along with the handout without anyone noticing.

Having considered the delivery of PowerPoint and poster presentation, we return to the topic of group presentations.

Delivery of group presentations

Working as part of a team is an important skill to develop during your nursing programme. Some of you will already have experienced working in teams and will be confident in negotiating and collaborating with others. If this is the case, you probably would have dealt with Jade in a very different way from Sam. For those of you who, like Sam, would have found Jade's behaviour unexpected, dealing with such situations will be challenging, especially if you lack self-confidence.

Group presentations are likely to be a feature of both summative and formative assessments within your nursing programme. Table 7.1 considers the differences between group and individual presentations.

Table 7.1 illustrates the fact that group presentations assess not only your understanding of an aspect of a topic, but also your ability to work effectively with others in the achievement of a common goal. Group assessments of this type also provide the opportunity for peers to share presentation skills and ideas. In comparison, individual presentations are focused on your ability to understand a topic and select out the key features for your presentation. Presentations need to communicate effectively these key factors through the use of a range of media. These might include a PowerPoint presentation, role play and poster presentation, for example.

Although Sam was left feeling let down and exploited by her first experience of a group presentation, she has learnt a valuable lesson about working with others early in her student journey. She has resolved to be clearer in future about the distribution of work when committing to group work, and to be more assertive when deadlines are not met. Her personal tutor had also directed her to the work of Johnson (2009) regarding guidance on resolving conflict.

Group presentation	Individual presentation
Jointly responsible for outcome of the presentation.	Solely responsible for outcome of the presentation.
Needs an overall understanding of topic.	Needs in-depth understanding of whole topic and in-depth understanding of your section.
Joint decision-making – need to negotiate and collaborate with others.	Individual decision-making – can work independently without a need to collaborate with others.
Offers additional presentation options, e.g. role play.	Limits use of some presentation options.
Benefits from sharing ideas and learning new techniques.	May limit experimentation in presentation options.

Table 7.1: Differences between group and individual presentations

Concept summary: Resolving conflict theory applied to scenario

By applying Johnson's approaches to conflict management (Johnson, 2009) Sam was helped to see how she might have behaved differently when communicating with Jade.

Withdrawing   This type of response ignores the problem in the hope that it will go away. By not challenging Jade over her behaviour, Sam's initial response to Jade's behaviour was to withdraw and fail to deal with the situation when problems began to emerge.

Forcing   People using this approach intend to meet their goals at all costs. Sam could see that this authoritarian approach reflects Jade's style of communication in order to meet her need to appear to have contributed to the group work. Her unexpected demand to introduce their section of the presentation caught Sam off guard and enabled Jade to achieve her goal.

Smoothing   Keeping the peace is the primary aim of this approach, and Sam could see this reflected in her behaviour. She did not want to 'make a fuss' and object to Jade's demands in front of her peers and tutor.

Compromising   This approach is constructive if it results in both parties being happy with the agreed compromise, and allowing some goals of each party to be achieved without too much damage to the relationship. This is the situation Sam will work towards in the future.

> *Problem solving/collaboration* Using this strategy, agreement benefits the people involved and enables negative feelings to be dissipated. It enables goals to be achieved and relationships maintained. Sam thinks that these last two approaches might have been the ones to use in developing her working relationship with Jade.
>
> In the scenario the style of conflict resolution was inappropriate, but each of the approaches outlined above can be effective dependent on the context of the communication.

In your professional career you will work in many teams. Some of these teams will prove cohesive, stimulating and exciting, while you may find that others work less effectively. Whatever the nature of the team you are working in, the most important aspect to consider is the impact the ineffective communication and conflict can have on the person receiving the service. In some situations this may prove a significant challenge, so learning to work effectively to produce a successful group presentation in university offers the opportunity to learn some of these lessons away from the practice arena.

Role play

Using role play as a means of presenting information is an alternative form of presentation that can be very powerful if done well and the chosen topic is suitable. For example, your group has been asked to present some aspect of professional communication, and you decide to use *assertive communication* as your topic. Acting out how a non-assertive communication can be changed into an assertive communication can be a very useful way of demonstrating how to be assertive.

There are some key factors to consider.

- Make sure your topic is suitable for role play.
- Develop an outline script and agree the purpose of each section of dialogue so that all students understand the gist of what needs to be said rather than learning the script verbatim. This is likely to result in a more spontaneous performance.
- Do not over-rehearse, as your performance may then be stilted and unconvincing.
- If the content of your role play is something that some in the audience may find distressing – for example, if your role play is about breaking bad news – it is important that the audience is aware of the topic in case someone has recently been the recipient of bad news and may become distressed as a result of witnessing the role play.

Using feedback from presentations

Sometimes the stress of giving a presentation can make students feel they have not done well. This may not be the view of the audience, however. Feedback from tutors will be provided for both formative and summative presentations, but you will not always be given formal feedback on your presentation from your fellow students. Be prepared to develop a simple feedback sheet you can give to your audience that will provide you with feedback on the best bits of your presentation and the areas where you could improve. You should find that this feedback will enable you to build your confidence for future successful presentations.

If you have no experience of using software packages such as PowerPoint or of poster production, then contact your university's student support/study centre for guidance and attend any workshops or online tutorials they can offer you.

Chapter summary

This chapter has identified the key points you need to consider to promote success in your formative or summative presentation. We have looked at three common types of presentation: PowerPoint presentations, poster presentations and group presentations. Each section has made links to the skills that delivering presentations can enable you to develop and how these skills can be used in practice.

Activities: brief outline answers

Activity 7.1: Communication and team working (page 92)

Sam discussed her experience with her personal tutor and developed a strategy to avoid a repetition of the experience with Jade.

- Be assertive from the outset and ask for a discussion on the ground rules that will guide the behaviour of group members, e.g. members will complete allocated work, attend agreed meetings. This would have allowed Sam to challenge Jade's behaviour when she deviated from the agreement and would have limited the amount of work she found herself doing.
- Agree with her sub-group which part of the presentation each person would contribute to.
- Indicate on each slide who has provided the information so that contribution is apparent.
- Be assertive and ensure that your work can stand alone and you present the information you have prepared.

Sam could also have disclosed the problems she was having to the rest of the group. Peer pressure may have encouraged Jade to contribute to her section of the group presentation and Sam may have benefited by the support of her peers.

Activity 7.2: Reflection and critical thinking (page 92)

- Ability to use technology to produce a presentation.
- Ability to speak audibly and concisely about a topic.
- Ability to talk to your slides using cue cards rather than reading from a prepared script.
- Ability to make good eye contact with the audience.
- Ability to smile at the audience (despite feeling nervous).
- Ability to demonstrate depth of knowledge and communicate information clearly.
- Ability to seek and receive feedback on performance and respond appropriately.

If you consider each of the bullet points above, you will see how developing these skills by delivering presentations can build skills that will enable you to effectively disseminate information to colleagues and people in your care.

Activity 7.3: Critical thinking and decision making (page 94)

As Jess is delivering this presentation to a small group of students she could choose to print out a handout of her PowerPoint presentation and use this to work through the content. As she is based in the clinical area Jess could opt to adapt her presentation to include activities for the students to undertake, for example, taking the pulse rate of a child and comparing the results with the normal range of pulse rate for the child's age group.

Introducing audience participation/activity can be a very effective way to gain and maintain audience attention.

Activity 7.5: Reflection and critical thinking (page 96)

This activity should reflect the final list of dos and don'ts initially set in Activity 7.4.

Dos	**Don'ts**
Do practise your presentation so that it flows and you can keep to time.	Don't fail to check room and equipment.
Do smile and make eye contact with your audience.	Don't leave preparation to the last minute.
Do speak clearly and strongly.	Don't read from a script.
Do make sure your audience can see and hear you.	Don't speak in a monotone.
Do clearly state purpose of presentation.	Don't fill the slides with too much text.
Do use cue cards.	Don't overuse animation and clip art.
Do keep to the point and know your subject so you can answer questions.	Don't use font and background colour that makes it difficult to read the slides.
Do seek feedback on your performance.	Don't overrun or fail to use all allocated time.

Further reading

Johnson, D (2009) *Reaching out: interpersonal effectiveness and self-actualisation*, 10th edition. Boston MA: Allyn & Bacon/Merrill.

This book is the source of information on conflict management.

McCray, J (ed) (2009) *Nursing and multi-professional practice*. London: Sage Publications.

Chapter 1 of this book offers insight into how professionals work together in practice.

Race, P, Brown, S and Smith, B (2005) *500 tips on assessment*. Abingdon: RoutledgeFalmer.

This book is written for tutors but may help students gain a greater understanding of the purpose of all assessments, including presentations.

Smale, B and Fowlie, J (2009) *How to succeed at university*. London: Sage Publications.

Chapter 7 of this book contains some useful sections on giving presentations.

Stein-Parbury, J (2005) *Patient and person*. Melbourne: Elsevier.

This excellent book on interpersonal skills has some interesting sections on conflict resolution and assertiveness in practice.

Useful websites

Access your university resources on presentations as they will provide guidance based on the criteria they use to assess presentations.

Chapter 8
Where to look for support with your assessments

Kay Hutchfield

NMC Standards for Pre-registration Nursing Education

This chapter will address the following competencies:

Domain 1: Professional values

8. All nurses must practise independently, recognising the limits of their competence and knowledge. They must reflect on these limits and seek advice from, or refer to other professionals where necessary.

Chapter aims

By the end of this chapter you should be able to:

*   identify a range of support resources you can access that will assist you in being successful in a range of assessments.

Introduction

In the previous chapters of this book you have been introduced to students who have been unsuccessful in their assessments and who have accessed a range of support services to improve their performance. This chapter aims to provide you with an overview of support services and resources available so that you can use these resources in advance of submitting your assessments, thus ensuring your assessments are likely to be successful.

It does not contain any scenarios or activities as it is designed to pull together the advice from all the chapters into one place for easy reference.

Student study support

All universities will have a student support/advice centre. Study skill is normally included as part of this service. Resources may be available in a number of formats.

- Workshops may be available on topics such as essay writing and examination techniques.
- Online tutorials, worksheets and additional information will be available instead of or to supplement workshops.
- Individual support will also be available if you have a specific problem or disability.

It is always best to check early on in your nursing programme what your student support centre has to offer so that you are familiar with what is on offer and can make a plan to use the resources you feel you may benefit from. For example, attending a workshop on critical analysis at the beginning of Year 2 will help you improve the level of analysis you develop in your work so that the quality of your work continues to improve.

If you are a student with a disability, a specific plan will be developed for you that will identify the support you need to be in place for you in university and in placement. These support plans will be reviewed on a regular basis.

IT support

This type of support will vary from institution to institution. It may be part of student support or be a separate service. Whatever the case, you need to discover what is available to you so that you have time to learn how to use any software you will need to use as part of your programme.

Help may be available as worksheets or as online tutorials.

Library

The support from your faculty/school librarian will be invaluable to you on your programme. They have specialist knowledge of the books, journals and other resources your university library holds for your subject. They are the ones most likely to be able to help you if your search for information on a topic draws a blank.

Your university library is also likely to offer library skills workshops or online tutorials. Developing your library skills will become increasingly important as you progress through your programme.

Make use of other resources available to you such as the NHS Evidence and RCN library to access additional library or study resources.

Assignment guidelines and learning outcomes

Assignment guidelines will direct you towards the format, word allowance and focus for your assignment. They will reflect the learning outcomes for the module/course for which the assignment is set. To be successful in any assessment it is essential that you focus clearly on the requirements of the learning outcomes and guidelines.

In addition to general study/library support and assessment guidelines, there are a number of individuals who will be an important source of support and advice for your assessments. However, it is important that before you seek help from these individuals you have made the effort to read your module/course handbook in addition to your assignment guidelines and learning outcomes. You will then be in a position to ask more focused and detailed questions of the individuals identified below.

The module/course leader

The name and contact details of the module/course leader will normally be found in the module/course handbook and VLE. They will be the person who has set the assignment and has academic responsibility for your learning, and will be the one to address your questions to about the assessment.

It may be advisable to email your question to the module/course leader rather than leave them to the end of a class.

You should avoid taking the advice of fellow students as they are not always right.

Your personal tutor

Your personal tutor will be reluctant to provide advice on an assessment for a module/course on which they do not teach or have never marked. It is always advisable to seek such advice from the module/course leader or seminar leader. However, your personal tutor can advise you on how to develop analysis in your work and will be aware of any plans you have made to improve your academic performance through your regular meetings.

Your personal tutor will know you as a person and something of your personal life. This is the person who will advise you if your personal life begins to impact negatively on your performance. They can direct you to sources of financial advice or counselling if this is the type of professional advice you need. Your personal tutor can also advise you on university regulations regarding interrupting your studies or how you might manage health issues.

Mentors

Your mentors will be very important support people in practice. Your relationship with your mentor should be a positive one, but to get the most out of the support they can offer it is essential that you develop an effective learning contract to discuss when you begin your placement. This will enable your mentor to be proactive on your behalf so that you gain the experience and learning opportunities you need to be successful in your practice assessments.

If you are experiencing difficulties, make sure you discuss them with your mentor so that they are in a position to be supportive and to seek assistance from the university if needed.

Link tutor

All your placements will be allocated a link tutor. Their role is to support both students and mentors in practice to promote high-quality supervision and positive practice assessment outcomes. If your performance falls below the expected standard at the formative stage of your practice assessment, the link tutor will attend a meeting with you and your mentor. Their role is to support you by ensuring that all university assessment procedures have been followed, that you are clear why your formative assessment has been unsuccessful and what you need to improve on if you are to meet your summative assessment.

Link tutors should be contacted if you do not have continuity despite raising the issue with the placement manager. Here they will act as a mediator for you and, if necessary, rearrange your shift patterns in order to achieve an appropriate level of mentorship for you.

Friends and family

Friends and family are the people who are likely to provide you with the most support during your programme. If your family and friends are supportive of your studies, then this can help to reduce stress at times when assessments are due.

If you have children, they may find it difficult to understand why you have to study. Try to set aside work to do when they are doing their homework so that you can work alongside each other if this is possible. Making time for family and friends and having fun is important in restoring your energy levels and allowing you to 'recharge your batteries'. Careful planning should allow you to build in time for this.

However, your strength and support may come from outside the family – perhaps from your religious community, from a university club or from playing sport. Whatever the source, it is important that you have a life outside study and placements that allows you to relax. Social activity will continue to be important once you have qualified as a way of reducing stress.

In conclusion, the most important thing to remember is that if you find yourself in difficulties, seek help early so that whatever the problem is, it does not escalate out of control; remember Nicky in Chapter 3. The consequences for Nicky would have been very different if she had told her link teacher about the problems she was experiencing completing her formative assessment.

> ### Chapter summary
>
> This chapter has drawn from all the preceding chapters in order to present a summary of the various support systems and resources that are available to help you be successful during your nursing programme. The most important point to emphasise is to make sure you are aware of all the support resources at your disposal at your university and, if needed, use them as soon as you realise a problem is likely to arise. In this way you are most likely to be successful in all the assessments in your programme.

Further reading

Hutchfield, K (2010) *Information skills for nursing*. Exeter: Learning Matters.

This book provides an introduction to professional development planning and the SBAR model of communication.

Price, B and Harrington, A (2010) *Critical thinking and writing for nursing students*. Exeter: Learning Matters.

If you need to improve your critical thinking and writing skills then this is the book for you.

Price, G and Maier, P (2007) *Effective study skills*. Harlow: Pearson Education Press.

This book has two useful chapters on improving your reading techniques and effective note-taking.

Reed, S (2011) *Success with your professional portfolio for nursing students*. Exeter: Learning Matters.

This book offers an introduction to developing a range of portfolios used in nursing.

Useful websites

www.evidence.nhs.uk/#

As a student in the NHS you are entitled to use The NHS Evidence site, which will be a useful resource to inform your studies.

www.palgrave.com/skills4study/studyskills/

This is an extensive study skills resource provided by Palgrave publications.

References

Benner, P (1984) *From novice to expert*. Menlo Park CA: Addison-Wesley.

Bloom, B S (ed) (1956) *Taxonomy of education objectives: Book 1 The cognitive domain*. London: Longman.

Bloomfield, J, Pegram, A and Jones, C (2010) *How to pass your OSCE: a guide to success in nursing and midwifery*. Harlow: Pearson Education.

Department of Health (2005) *Mental Capacity Act 2005*. Available at: www.legislation.gov.uk/ukpga/2005/9/contents/enacted (accessed November 2011).

Department of Health (2007) *Essence of care: patient focused benchmarks for clinical governance*. London: NHS Modernisation Agency.

Dougherty, L and Lister, S (eds) (2011) *The Royal Marsden Hospital manual of clinical procedures*, 8th Student edition. Chichester: Wiley-Blackwell.

Howatson-Jones, L (2010) *Reflective practice in nursing*. Exeter: Learning Matters.

Hutchfield, K (2010) *Information skills for nursing students*. Exeter: Learning Matters.

Johnson, D (2009) *Reaching out: interpersonal effectiveness and self-actualisation*, 10th edition. Boston MA: Allyn & Bacon/Merrill.

NICE (National Institute for Health and Clinical Excellence) (2003) *Infection control: prevention of healthcare-associated infection in primary and community care* (CG2). Available at: http://guidance.nice.org.uk/CG2 (accessed 8 March 2012).

NICE (2007) *Acutely ill patients in hospital: recognition of and response to acute illness in adults in hospital, NICE clinical guideline 50*. London: NICE. Accessed at: www.nice.org.uk/guidance/CG50.

NMC (Nursing and Midwifery Council) (2008) *The code: Standards of conduct, performance and ethics for nurses and midwives*. London: NMC.

NMC (2010a) *Strategic context report*. Available at www.nmc-uk.org/About-us/Our-strategic-vision/.

NMC (2010b) *Standards for pre-registration nursing education*. Available at: http://standards.nmc-uk.org/Pages/Welcome.aspx.

NMC (2010c) *Essential skills clusters for pre-registration nursing education*. Available at: http://standards.nmc-uk.org/Documents/Annexe3_%20ESCs_16092010.pdf.

NMC (2011a) *Guidance for students*. London: NMC. Available at: www.nmc-uk.org/Students/Guidance-for-students/.

NMC (2011b) *The prep handbook*. Available at: www.nmc-uk.org/Educators/Standards-for-education/The-Prep-handbook/.

Nulty, D D, Mitchell, M L, Jeffery, C A, Henderson, A and Groves, M (2011) Best practice guidelines for the use of OSCEs: maximising value for student learning. *Nurse Education Today* 31: 145–51.

Price, B and Harrington, A (2010) *Critical thinking and writing for nursing students*. Exeter: Learning Matters.

QAA (Quality Assurance Agency) (2006) *Code of practice for the assurance of academic quality and standards in higher education. Section 6: Assessment of students*. Available at www.qaa.ac.uk/AssuringStandardsAndQuality/code-of-practice/Pages/default.aspx.

QAA (2008a) *Framework for higher education qualifications in England and Wales*. Available at www.qaa.ac.uk/Publications/InformationAndGuidance/Pages/The-framework-for-higher-education-qualifications-in-England-Wales-and-Northern-Ireland.aspx.

QAA (2008b) *Subject benchmark statements: health studies*. Available at www.qaa.ac.uk/Publications/Information AndGuidance/Pages/Subject-benchmark-statement-Health-studies.aspx.

Reed, S (2011) *Success with your professional portfolio for nursing students*. Exeter: Learning Matters.

Rushforth, H (2007) Objective Structured Clinical Examination (OSCE): review of literature and implications for nursing education. *Nurse Education Today* 27: 481–90.

UNICEF (2006) Behind closed doors. Available at: www.unicef.org/media/files/BehindClosedDoors.pdf.

Watson, R, Stimpson, A, Topping, A and Porock, D (2002) Clinical competence in assessment in nursing: a systematic review of the literature. *Journal of Advanced Nursing* 39 (5): 421–31.

Index

22664517R00070

Made in the USA
Middletown, DE
06 August 2015